T0361937

Aleen Cust

Originally published in 1990, this book is a valuable contribution to the history of the veterinary profession in Great Britain and Ireland. Connie Ford's book is a reminder of the great social changes that have taken place since Aleen Cust was born in 1868. When Aleen Cust entered the New Veterinary College, Edinburgh in 1895, and was later refused permission to sit the examinations of the Royal College of Veterinary Surgeons, no British woman had the vote. New a new generation of veterinarians will find this account of the life and times of a truly remarkable woman a revelation.

Aleen Cust Veterinary Surgeon

Britain's First Woman Vet

Connie M. Ford

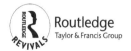

First published in 1990 by Biopress Ltd

This edition first published in 2024 by Routledge
4 Park Square, Milton Park, Abingdon, Oxon, OX14 4RN
and by Routledge
605 Third Avenue, New York, NY 10158.

Routledge is an imprint of the Taylor & Francis Group, an informa business

© 1990 Biopress Ltd

The right of Connie M. Ford to be identified as the author of this work has been asserted
by her in accordance with sections 77 and 78 of the Copyright, Designs and Patents Act
1988.

All rights reserved. No part of this book may be reprinted or reproduced or utilised in
any form or by any electronic, mechanical, or other means, now known or hereafter
invented, including photocopying and recording, or in any information storage or
retrieval system, without permission in writing from the publishers.

ISBN 13: 978-1-032-78792-3 (hbk)
ISBN 13: 978-1-003-48997-9 (ebk)
ISBN 13: 978-1-032-78960-6 (pbk)
Book DOI 10.4324/9781003489979

Aleen Cust, Veterinary Surgeon

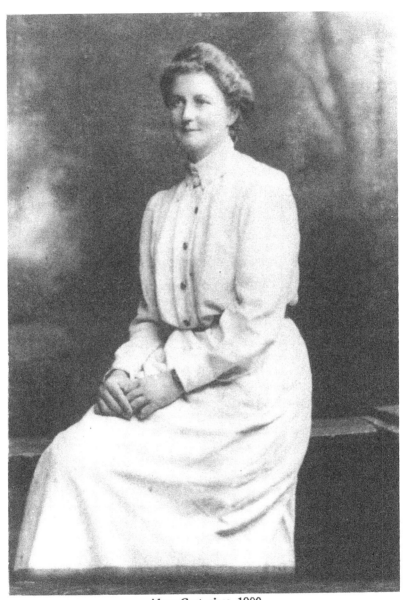

Aleen Cust, circa. 1900

Aleen Cust
Veterinary Surgeon

Britain's First Woman Vet

Connie M. Ford

M.B.E., M.R.C.V.S.

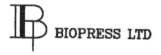 BIOPRESS LTD

© Biopress Ltd 1990

All rights reserved. No part of this publication may be reproduced, stored in a retrieval system, or transmitted, in any form or by any means, electronic, mechanical, photocopying, recording or otherwise, without the prior permission of the copyright owner.

ISBN 0-948-737-11-5

PUBLISHED BY:

Biopress Ltd.
`The Orchard´
Clanage Road
Bristol
BS3 2JX
England

British Library Cataloguing in Publication Data

Ford, Connie M.
    Aleen Cust, veterinary surgeon.
    1. Great Britain, Veterinary medicine. Cust, Aleen
    I. Title
    636.089092

    ISBN 0-948737-11-5

Printed in Great Britain by View Publications (Bristol) Ltd. at Wickwar, Gloucestershire

Dedication

To all veterinary students, everywhere,
especially the women.

Acknowledgements

So many people have helped me with this book that it is impossible to list them all. I have had generous hospitality in out of the way places - and even in central London - during my travels in Great Britain and Ireland in pursuit of my researches. I have had access to private archives, and introductions to helpful people, and I have delved in a great variety of libraries. Chief of these was the RCVS Wellcome Library, where Miss Horder and her staff were incredibly patient and helpful.

Miss Gwynedd Lloyd, CVO, DL, and Commander A. G. Skipwith, who are related to Miss Cust, and Captain Francis Widdrington and Captain A. J. Baker-Cresswell, who are grand-children of the man who became Aleen's guardian on her father's death, have all given me invaluable help and information.

Among professional colleagues Pat Hewlett (nee Williams) was a mine of information and encouragement, and I have had technical help with the script from several senior people who had the knowledge of horse practice which I so sadly lacked. I had fascinating conversations with Mrs Taylor (nee Knight), the second British woman veterinary surgeon, who followed close on Aleen's heels in 1923, and I have learned much from Iain Pattison and his own exemplary books of veterinary history. I also had help from literary friends outside the profession who could check me if I became too technical for the general reader, and from Roger Renshaw who reproduced the photographs for me from a great variety of sources and standardised their format.

I wish to thank the Society of Women Veterinary Surgeons for financial assistance in publishing this book.

Finally, I am indebted to my late sister, Edith Ford, who invented the verb `to Cust´ and was a most patient listener during those times when I could talk of nothing else.

Connie M. Ford

Table of Contents

List of Illustrations

Foreword

"There is no history; only biography."

Ralph Waldo Emerson

Whether or not one agrees with Waldo Emerson, there is no doubt that Connie Ford's biography of Aleen Cust is a valuable contribution to the history of the veterinary profession in Great Britain and Ireland. It is published at a time when, paradoxically, although the Republic of Ireland has become more closely linked with the United Kingdom within the European Community, the special relationship between the profession in the Republic and the Royal College of Veterinary Surgeons has, to our mutual regret, been severed.

Connie Ford's book is a reminder of the great social changes that have taken place since Aleen Cust was born in 1868. Not only was society then completely male oriented (indeed, male dominated) but very few women supported the women's rights movements. When Aleen Cust entered the New Veterinary College, Edinburgh as a student in October 1895, and was later refused permission to sit the examinations of the Royal College of Veterinary Surgeons, no British woman had the vote. Indeed, when she was eventually registered as the first woman Member of the Royal College of Veterinary Surgeons in 1922, married women, women householders and women university graduates had had the right to vote for only four years; and even then, only if they were over 30 years of age. Not until 1928 did women have the same voting rights as men.

Connie Ford gives us a glimpse of life in the British Isles at the turn of the century and almost up to the Second World War. The attitudes of the aristocracy, into which Aleen Cust was born, are given an airing; as are the strange views about women held by most members of the veterinary profession at the time. Life, especially in rural Ireland before the advent of the motor car, is depicted as quite idyllic, except for the rural poor.

New generations of veterinarians, especially women, will find this account of the life and times of a truly remarkable woman a revelation. We should all feel grateful that so many eccentrics like Aleen Cust, with their determination and strength of character, have always enriched our profession by their presence.

Those of us who have known of Connie Ford's passion for her subject and listened to her speak about her favourite veterinary surgeon are delighted to see her book in print at last, giving others a chance to share our pleasure and her enthusiasm.

H. E. Carter, MRCVS
Past President of the RCVS

Introduction

In the early years of the twentieth century a tall handsome woman might have been seen riding purposefully about the Irish countryside on a white Arab stallion.

This was Aleen Cust, an English aristocrat, and the first British woman to become a veterinary surgeon. She was fully trained, at the New Edinburgh Veterinary College, and a highly successful practitioner, but officially she did not exist. The Royal College of Veterinary Surgeons, governing body of the profession in Britain, had refused to let her sit for any of their examinations. This meant that she could not even call herself a veterinary surgeon as she was not on their Register. Yet she persisted in her chosen career, and was loved and respected for miles around.

She came to Roscommon in 1900 as assistant to William Byrne, a rising young practitioner in the small country town of Athleague. She was soon independent of him, but his continued friendship helped her to gain acceptance from the other veterinary surgeons in the district, and after his death in 1910 she took over the whole practice. She even held a post as inspector for the Galway County Council to administer the Diseases of Animals Act, despite the strong disapproval of the RCVS in London.

During the 1914-18 war she went to France. Although desperately short of veterinary surgeons the Army disdained to accept her services officially, but she probably did quite a lot unofficially while ostensibly working for the YMCA.

After the war an Act of Parliament made it illegal to bar women from any profession merely on account of their sex, and in 1922 she was allowed to sit the final examination of the RCVS, and was awarded their Diploma and put on the Register. By this time she was a greyhaired lady of fifty-four, and her health was not good, so she retired to a village in the New Forest, where she bred dogs, attended the meetings of the local Veterinary Association, and basked in the belated recognition of her powers.

To the women students, only admitted to the London Veterinary College in 1927, she was a legend and an example, her name a private battle cry in their darkest moments. If they got on so much better than the old men of the RCVS had predicted, it was the trail blazing of this remarkable woman that had eased their path.

CHAPTER I

Childhood in Tipperary

*"... as I was green and carefree, famous among the barns
About the happy yard and singing as the farm was home ..."*

Dylan Thomas

Aleen Isabel Cust was born into a very distinguished family. Her mother was a grand-daughter of the Earl of Bradford, and became a Woman of the Bed-chamber to Queen Victoria. Her father was a grandson of Lord Brownlow, and godson to Leopold, King of the Belgians. Her father's mother, an expert horsewoman, was very fond of cats and wrote a small book on their diseases and management. Other relatives include a speaker of the House of Commons in the eighteenth century, a Dean of York, an art historian who became Director of the National Portrait Gallery, and a military historian who was Master of Ceremonies to Queen Victoria. A passage in her grandfather's Will suggests some connection with the family of Sir Isaac Newton, but the precise nature of this is not clear. Of her brothers, one died young, but not before he had been appointed as a page to Queen Victoria. Of the others, one was in the Navy and became Equerry to King George Vth, one joined the Army and later managed part of Lord Brownlow's estate, and the fourth, despite poor health, seems to have been interested in engineering and photography.

Aleen's father, Leopold Cust, at the age of thirty-two, married Charlotte Bridgeman, the daughter of a Vice-Admiral, and within a few years he was living in Ireland employed as `agent´ by a Mr Smith-Barry, afterwards Lord Barrymore, who owned much land in the county of Tipperary. Smith-Barry was not popular in the district, and Leopold's work must have been difficult and thankless, but the financial rewards probably made it worth-while. He lived some miles south-east of the town of Tipperary at Cordangan Manor, a beautiful country house set in spacious grounds with meadows, woods, and a small river. Here, on 7th February 1868, Aleen was born. Leopold registered her name as `Aileen´ but she always signed herself `Aleen´. He registered the child's

1

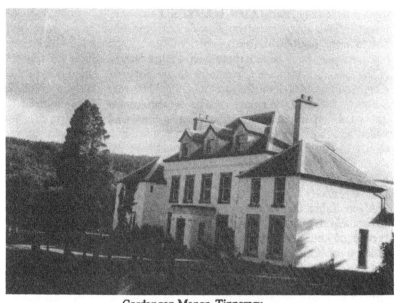

Cordangan Manor, Tipperary

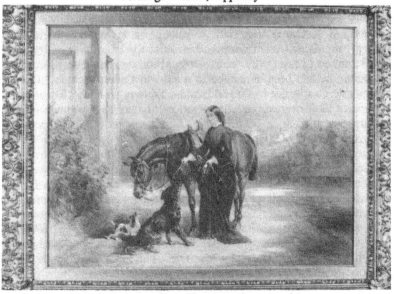

Lady Isabel Cust, Aleen's mother, as a girl

2

mother as merely `Isabel Cust' but her full name was `Charlotte Sobieske Isabel'. This abbreviation on Aleen's birth certificate might have been due to haste, excitement, or merely her father's impatience of ceremony, but there may have been a more deep-seated reason. Sobieske was one of the names of Princess Clementine Maria Sobieske, grand-daughter of King John Sobieski of Poland, who in 1719 married James Francis Stewart, the `Old Pretender'. The wealth of her dowry played an important part in maintaining the court in France of the `King over the water' and their son was Bonnie Prince Charlie. If any of the Bridgeman family had Jacobite sympathies they would have had to keep very quiet about it, but many aristocratic families did feel a certain nostalgia for the Stewarts. Perhaps by 1835, when Aleen's mother was born, Culloden was sufficiently long ago for her father, Vice-Admiral the Hon. Charles Orlando Bridgeman, to pay unobtrusive tribute to his namesake by calling his daughter `Sobieske'. Leopold, a staunch pillar of the Protestant Church of Ireland, may well have been irritated by his father-in-law's romantic notions and deliberately ignored the name. In any case she was always called `Isabel' by her own family.

Leopold is a rather shadowy figure who seems to have shunned the limelight of the court that played so freely on the rest of his family. Nevertheless in 1874 Queen Victoria appointed him one of her `Gentleman Ushers'. This did not involve him in regular duties, and he only rarely had to attend court. So his children were reared in rustic peace, and young Aleen rampaged at will in the beautiful countryside, with horses and dogs to her heart's content and three older brothers to rub shoulders with. Another brother arrived when she was two, and sister Ursula was born seven years later when she was nine. By this time her mother was forty-two, and this sixth child may have been somewhat unexpected.

Aleen was a big girl with good strong features, red hair, and the strong will and temper that often goes with it. She was warm-hearted and plucky, with an impish sense of humour. Judging by her subsequent exploits she must have enjoyed rude health, and those first ten years of her life were probably as carefree and exhilarating as all children's lives should be.

It was just before her tenth birthday, on 14th January, 1878, that her grandfather, old Sir Edward Cust, died at his home in London at the age of eighty-six. It is doubtful if she knew him personally, but his death made an important change in the family, as Leopold inherited the baronetcy and most of his father's fortune of some £18,000. How far it would have altered his manner of life it is difficult to judge.

3

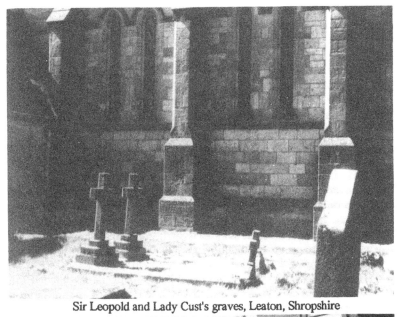

Sir Leopold and Lady Cust's graves, Leaton, Shropshire

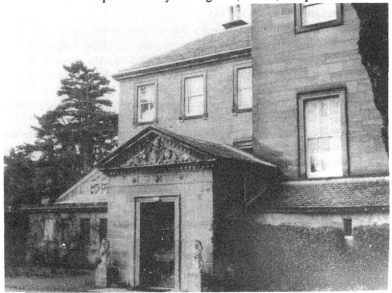

Newton Hall, Northumberland

4

He continued in his employment, but by the time his friends and servants had got used to calling him `Sir Leopold´ he was beginning to suffer from gout, the characteristic plague of the affluent in Victorian society.

Then, in March, tragedy struck. Some five or six miles north of Cordangan Manor was a small convent, and the Mother Superior decided it would be a nice arrangement if they could have a little graveyard specially built near by so that when they died the nuns could be buried close to their home and place of work and worship. This was done, and the first nun to die after it was completed was the sister of the priest of that parish. He officiated at the funeral and she was duly buried with all the appropriate rites. Soon afterwards Sir Leopold rode up. He had known nothing about the building of the graveyard and he was much incensed that such a thing should have been done on Smith-Barry's land without the landlord's knowledge or consent. He therefore upbraided the priest and said the nun should not have been buried there without his permission. The priest looked him in the eye and said, "Sir Leopold, will you put your leg on the grave".

He did so, and immediately he felt a sharp pain all down his leg. He got home with some difficulty, and was dead before morning, at the early age of forty-six. The story of his death has passed into the local folklore as a spectacular instance of God's vengeance on a hard and impious English heretic. It was described a hundred-and-three years later, by a retired farm worker on the estate, as vividly as if he had personally witnessed it. To a medically trained mind it seems a good clinical description of an embolism of the iliac artery, precipitated by a sudden rise in blood pressure. The death certificate gives `Heart failure, associated with gout´ as the cause of death, but no amount of medical testimony would have convinced the Roman Catholic peasantry of 1878 that the spiritual power of the priest had not been involved. Moreover many people heartily approved this particular act of retribution. Sir Leopold's death was reported in the *"Tipperary Free Press and Clonmel Advertiser"* as follows:

> "Sir Leopold Cust, agent over the extensive property in this country of Mr Arthur H. Smith-Barry, died suddenly on last Sunday. We regret very much to learn that on receipt of the intelligence in Tipperary Town, where Mr Cust was unfortunately very unpopular, the event was made the occasion of a very unseemly demonstration."

5

With commendable restraint no further details were given, and it was left to the reader's imagination to guess at the shocking behaviour of the inhabitants of Tipperary that Sunday evening.

For Lady Cust, living with her children in the stately home that went with the job, it must have been an even more devastating blow than most bereavements. Sir Leopold had specified in his Will that he was to be buried near wherever he died, and that the funeral should be as plain as possible, the cost not to exceed fifteen pounds. Lady Cust, tormented by the rumours, had other ideas, and Leopold's body was crated and sent to Cork, from where it was shipped to England and buried in Leaton churchyard in Shropshire. She herself took the children to England with all speed, and when Leopold's Will was proved, her address was given as Sansaw Hall, Shrewsbury, Salop. There are detailed records of this pleasant old house going back to the eighteenth century, but there is no mention in these of the Custs having lived there. Nor does there seem to be evidence of their living anywhere else, although an aristocratic widow with five children (Charles being already in the Navy) should have been fairly conspicuous in local society. Possibly they stayed for long periods with one or another of Lady Cust's sisters, or with her widowed mother, all of whom lived in Shropshire.

For Aleen, childhood had ended with brutal abruptness. Wrenched from the only home she had known, she found herself in a strange country among strangers. Her eldest brother, barely fourteen years old, was now Sir Charles Cust, and she herself was Miss Cust, the elder daughter of a stricken family.

A father, particularly in Victorian times, was naturally the lynchpin of the household, and the bond between Leopold and his first-born daughter may well have been very strong. She was now ten years old, too old to be insulated from the gossip of grooms and servants, and from the counsels of her elders. To the grief and shock of her sudden loss was added bewilderment at the wild talk about the nature of Leopold's death and the controversy preceding it. The alien aspects of Ireland, with the clash of religion and class - barely noticed till now - were suddenly thrust into her consciousness. Perhaps her level-headed understanding of the Irish in later life came from having to think these things out under the pressure of violent emotion at the age of ten.

One provision of Leopold's Will was most faithfully carried out. In a codicil dated 8th November, 1867, three months before Aleen was born, he wrote:

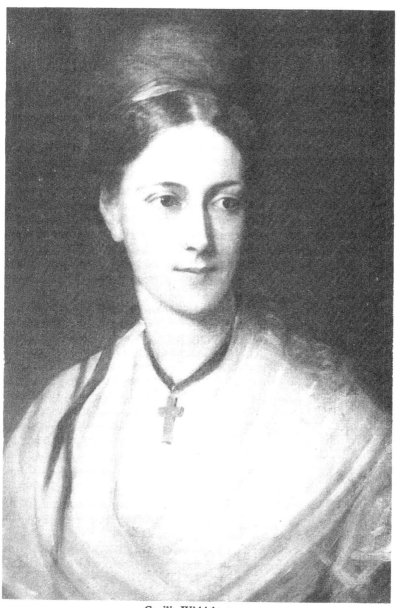

Cecilia Widdrington

"I appoint my wife to be the guardian of my children in conjunction with my friend Shallcross Fitzherbert Widdrington, of Newton Hall, Northumberland."

Evidently the two men were close friends, and as the Widdringtons were distantly related to the Smith-Barrys in Ireland, Major Widdrington may have had something to do with Leopold's appointment in Tipperary. He remained a firm friend to these fatherless children, several of whom often stayed with him and his wife at Newton Hall. Charles and Aleen seem to have been particularly frequent visitors, and they became very friendly with the Widdrington children. Newton Hall is a beautiful house high up on the Northumbrian moors above the village of Felton. It is sheltered by woods, which open out to the East to give a picturesque view of a lake, and in the distance the sea, about seven miles away. Major Widdrington was five years younger than Sir Leopold, and lived on to his ninety-second year, dying in December 1917, so the friendship was a long one, and highly valued. His wife, Cecilia, who died in 1938, kept a diary, much treasured by her grandchildren, one of whom still lives at Newton Hall, and this diary makes frequent mention of Aleen Cust.

In her Will, Aleen describes Dorothy, the eldest child of the Widdringtons, as `the greatest friend of my life´ and she left money to the British Trust for Ornithology in memory of her. Dorothy married Viscount Grey of Falloden in 1885, but she died in 1906 and there were no children. The Widdringtons lived in quiet comfort, hunted and rode with as much enthusiasm as Aleen herself, and cultivated their very beautiful gardens. Major Shallcross Fitzherbert - `Fitz´ to his wife - had the thoughtful face of a scholar, according to a portrait still at Newton Hall. He may well have been a steadying influence on the impetuous Aleen, but he also positively encouraged her ambition to do something more with her life than the average Victorian female of good family. At one time she tried nursing in the London Hospital, but found she disliked it, and felt much more sympathy for animals.

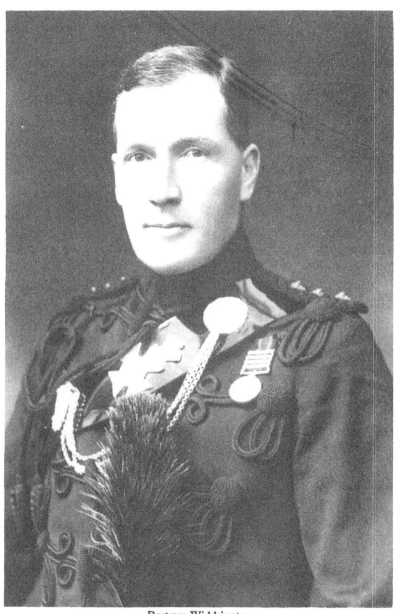

Bertram Widdrington

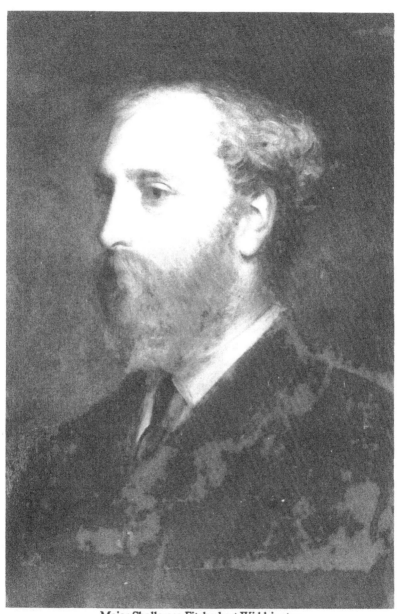

Major Shallcross Fitzherbert Widdrington

10

CHAPTER II

The Controversial Student

"Thou large-brained woman and large-hearted man"

Elizabeth Barrett Browning - `To George Sand´

In *Who's Who* Miss Cust's education was described as `private´. It is interesting to speculate on the influences that nurtured her lively mind to the point where she could embark upon the veterinary course. She both rode and drove from babyhood, so that any intellectual progress was matched from the start by practical skills. However conventional her lessons may have been, someone taught her the art of studying and learning, and managed to do this without damping down the natural curiosity that goes with and feeds on sharp observation. In Ireland, when they were little, she was probably taught with her brothers and this could have stimulated an interest in the natural sciences beyond what might otherwise have been considered suitable for a young lady.

By the time their father died her brother Charles was already in the Royal Navy, but Brownlow and Percy both went eventually to Wellington College. This is a Public School set up to provide education for the children of men in the Services, and Sir Leopold's children qualified by reason of his service as a lieutenant in the North Salop Yeomanry from 1867 to 1873. However, Brownlow did not go to the College till 1881, when he was sixteen years old, and as no other school is mentioned in his extensive obituary in the *Shrewsbury Chronicle* of 1893 it is likely that he was previously taught at home. The third brother, Leopold, was delicate from birth and did not go to Wellington College at all, although Percy, the youngest, went there in 1884. It would seem likely, then, that all three brothers were educated at home, presumably by a tutor, at least until 1881, and Leopold for a longer period. Lady Cust was deemed by her wealthier relatives to be in straitened circumstances, and she may well have economised by letting Aleen share a tutor with her brothers instead of having a separate governess for her. This could mean that she had a far more liberal education than most girls of that period.

11

If her reading was unrestricted she could have plunged into the heady fermentation of ideas that characterised the latter part of the nineteenth century. Her passion for animals would have laid her wide open to the work of Darwin and Huxley, and the interplay of ideas with her brothers would have been a further stimulus. By the time all the brothers but Leopold had left home she was already under the influence of the Widdringtons. Cecilia Widdrington was a `free thinker' and may have deliberately encouraged her to question her mother's conventions. In any case Aleen could hardly have escaped the excitement of the new ideas about women's emancipation. Florence Nightingale had already revolutionised the Nursing profession. Miss Buss and Miss Beale were battling in the cause of women's education, and Elizabeth Garrett Anderson had become a doctor. In 1889 a French woman doctor had taken the veterinary course in France and set up in practice in Paris. How much Aleen knew of these individuals is uncertain, but in only a few years time the suffragettes were effectively to shatter the myth of women's docile passivity.

Yet it is quite likely that the major factor in deciding Aleen on a veterinary career was friendship with veterinary surgeons and close observation of them at their work. `Vets' are tolerant and kindly people, on the whole, and the frantic opposition of some of them to the entry of women into their profession was the sort of aberration that occurs when men feel threatened by the unknown. Meanwhile, within reasonable limits, the customer was always right. When the customer was a young and beautiful girl who was exceptionally `good with animals' and took a highly intelligent interest in all aspects of their work, most men would bask in the eyes of such a good listener. Some may even have said jokingly that she `ought' to have been a `vet' herself, all the time being securely convinced that such a thing was impossible.

It might have remained a wild dream but for a family tragedy which gave Aleen an unexpected windfall. In the summer of 1893 Orlando, as her second-eldest brother was usually called, died very suddenly after a few days illness with meningitis. He had left home for employment by Lord Brownlow, a kinsman of his father, to manage some estates near Ellesmere, Shropshire. He was a popular young man, only twenty-seven years old, and a frequent visitor to Weston Park, the imposing estate of his cousin, the Earl of Bradford. He was unmarried, and he had made no Will, so it fell to brother Charles, as head of the family, to administer his estate of some £3,000. According to the law at that time it would have been divided in equal portions between his mother and his four brothers and sisters. Aleen's portion would therefore have been about £600 - enough for a few years of independence if she were careful.

Lady Cust was at that time a Woman of the Bed-chamber to Queen Victoria, and it is unlikely she would have approved of any unconventional behaviour, yet in 1894 Aleen went to Edinburgh, determined to become a veterinary surgeon. In later life she was increasingly estranged from her family, and it was Major Widdrington who escorted her to Edinburgh, found her suitable lodgings, and gave her the moral support that her family denied her. She managed to support herself in Edinburgh as a student for the next five years. In a letter to the *Veterinary Record* in 1934 she said that in 1898 she was "...half starving on six shillings and sixpence a week, eating only one solid meal a day at a cost of five pence in company with the newspaper boys of Edinburgh, my only other meal being of raw oatmeal with hot water poured over it... I was living in an attic in winter with no fire, and when too cold to work any more I used to go out after dark into the quiet back streets and run to get warm enough to sleep..." Of such stuff are pioneers made!

She spent the first year in Edinburgh gaining sufficient paper qualifications for entry to the veterinary course. This was the same as for medical students, and presumably she would have studied with these at Edinburgh University.

How she actually got herself into the veterinary college is not known, but her long remembered gratitude to Principal William Williams suggests that she managed to convince him of her suitability, after which his faith in her never wavered. He was originally principal of the older `Dick´ Edinburgh veterinary college (so called after its founder, William Dick), but in 1873 he had resigned and set up a rival college called the New Veterinary College, Edinburgh, which was eventually moved to Liverpool University. During the years when both colleges were in Edinburgh there was keen competition between them, and this may have facilitated her entry if Professor Williams thought that her brilliance, and the novelty of being the first woman student, would ultimately add to his prestige.

She registered as a student under the name of `A. I. Custance´, presumably to spare her mother's susceptibilities if there should be any undue publicity. The choice of pseudonym is interesting as besides the convenience of its being so close to her real name, it was the name of a very famous jockey. Henry Custance, born in 1842, rode three Derby winners and many others, his last in 1879. He continued to be a prominent figure in both English and Belgian race courses, being starter to the Belgian Jockey Club and deputy starter to the British Jockey Club,

13

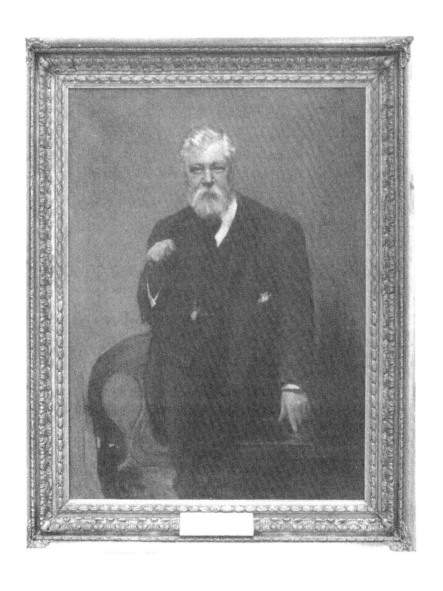

Principal William Williams, FRCVS

and he hunted regularly with the Quorn and Cottesmore. The girl who adored horses and was well-connected in the Shires may possibly have been introduced to him, and she would certainly have known the name. He was probably a hero of her youth, and in her wilder moments she might even have wished to emulate him. Being called `Miss Custance´ in Edinburgh would be a private joke and a boost to her morale.

A veterinary college in the nineties was a rough and hectic place. Major A. Spreull was a fellow-student of Miss Cust in 1896. In 1935 he became President of the Scottish Metropolitan Veterinary Association, and in his presidential address gave us this glimpse of his student days:

> "The Principal was perhaps the finest old practical veterinary surgeon of that time, and a wonderful teacher. When on the subject of lameness his practical demonstrations in class, when he hobbled around in his white spats and imitated each particular lameness, can never be forgotten."

Among his young staff was Professor O. Charnock Bradley, a famous anatomist who became Principal of the older `Dick´ Veterinary College in 1911. Major Spreull recalled that in 1897 Bradley was

> "just beginning to impress his authority and to repress the muscle fights and chaos of the New Veterinary College dissecting room, where the studious young anatomists had to work under a barrage of fascia, while cricket enthusiasts, armed with a dry forelimb and scapula, defended themselves from all comers."

The term `muscle fights´ referred to pitched battles in which the missiles were chunks of discarded meat from the carcasses under dissection. `Fascia´ is the membranous covering of these muscles, which has to be dissected away to reveal the detailed structure. At the Royal Veterinary College, London, these goings-on were known as `meat fights´ and were strictly forbidden, but they went on clandestinely at least until 1930. By that time the small corps of women students simply huddled in a corner, while the men gave them all their watches and fountain pens for safe keeping until the fracas was over, but when Miss Cust was all alone in the Edinburgh bear garden it must have been much more daunting. This was hinted at by Major F. J. Taylor, of Oxford, who was also a fellow-student of Aleen, and spoke of her at a meeting of the

Southern Counties Veterinary Association soon after her death in 1937. He said:

> "She sat next to me in class during the first and second term. She was always a most diligent student, and a very pleasing person to know, and she carried out her arduous studies under very great difficulties. Perhaps there are few of you here who realise the difference between the life of the veterinary student in those days and what it is today. Miss Cust was the lady pioneer of our profession, and you can well imagine that in those days it was very difficult for her to establish any position of respect, because men of a certain type were inclined to jeer at her, and thought she ws extremely foolish to think of joining a profession like ours, which at that time was essentially a man's job. But she maintained her position and eventually gained the great respect of everyone, and became, as you know, an extremely brilliant practitioner and student, being first in all her classes."

Miss Cust's apprenticeship with four lively brothers probably enabled her to hold her own, even with Edinburgh veterinary students.

It was in April 1897 that the first shots were exchanged in a sporadic warfare that was to last for the next thirty years. Some will say it is still going on, but the positions have changed so much that present day battles are quite different.

The earliest mention of it came in the report of one of the quarterly meetings of the Council of the RCVS. The Council, the governing body of the profession, was composed of veterinary surgeons elected by the whole profession. Some were in general practice in different parts of the country, some were professors at one or another of the various veterinary colleges, and some were in the Army, attached to cavalry regiments. In theory anyone on the Register was eligible for nomination to Council, but in practice they would all be senior members, many very eminent in their respective spheres. The detailed business of the Council was carried on by various committees, appointed by the Council from among themselves. One such committee was responsible for organising the professional examinations, twice a year, at the colleges of London, Edinburgh, and Glasgow. They also evaluated the certificates of general education which students had to produce before commencing their first year studies. At this meeting, on 14th April 1897, Mr W. J. Mulvey, chairman of the Examination Committee, reported that they had been asked to consider an application from Miss A. I. Custance, "she having

16

produced the necessary education certificate for admission to the first professional examination", but they did not consider they had the power to admit women to that examination, and had referred the matter to the solicitor.

When the Chairman's report had been duly adopted, Professor W. O. Williams, of the New Edinburgh College where Aleen was a student, asked for the Solicitor's report. Mr George Thatcher, Solicitor to the RCVS, was a middle-aged man, wily, conventional, and a master of circumlocution. In his ensuing peroration he quoted at length from the Veterinary Surgeon's Charter of 1844, and cited several cases of a "somewhat analogous nature". His report may be fairly summarised by saying that although there was no logical reason why she should not be admitted, the fact that in the preceding fifty-three years no woman had been admitted meant that `usage will now preclude her`. However, he was anxious to hedge his bets, and he "put this view with great diffidence, and would respectfully suggest" that the opinion of their Counsel be taken.

Mr Mulvey observed: "The question is undoubtedly one of very great importance, and I therefore move that Counsel's opinion is taken in the matter and acted upon" and this was seconded. Professor Pritchard asked what Counsel's fee would be, and on being told that it would b e two guineas, said; "Then I do not think the game is worth the candle, and I should let Miss Custance go in for the examination". Whether this was genuine thrift or a surreptitious attempt to help her we shall never know, but the Council were nervous of such a simple solution. Professor Williams pointed out that it was only a month before the examination, and that "a good many members of the Council knew a year ago that Miss Custance was going up for the examination". Mr Mulvey interposed, saying "Perhaps you will allow me to explain that, as chairman of the Examination Committee, I had no idea whatsoever that the name of `Custance` which appeared was that of a woman". Professor Williams pointed to the entry of women into the medical profession, and suggested that they might be guided by this, but the lawyer said that the case was quite different. The medical profession had decided according to its own Charters and Acts, and the veterinary profession should make an independent judgement. This touched a raw nerve, as the veterinary profession was always jealous of the higher standing with the public that the medical profession appeared to enjoy, even in matters concerning animal diseases, where the veterinary surgeon's knowledge of comparative pathology was inevitably superior.

17

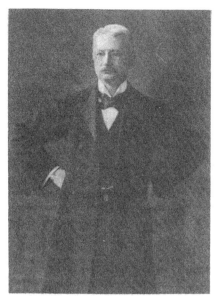

Professor William Owen Williams, FRCVS, FRSE

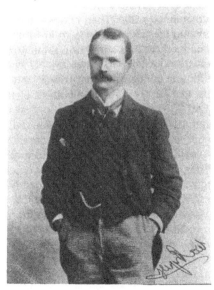

William Augustine Byrne, MRCVS

18

The Army had by now found its voice, and Veterinary Col. Lambert, a veteran of the Zulu War and several others, said: "As this is one of the most important things ever brought up before the Council since I have had anything to do with it, may I ask whether the opinion of the standing Counsel of the College is final and binding as far as our action goes?". The President said the resolution before them was to that effect, but several Council members said they would like to discuss Counsel's opinion before acting upon it. Professor Williams moved that they allow Miss Custance to sit the examination, and Professor Pritchard of London seconded this, but Mr Dollar, a Councillor who loved argument and was instinctively against the merest whiff of innovation, urged caution. "To take Counsel's opinion binds us to do nothing, while the other course establishes a precedent". They voted against letting her sit, and agreed to take Counsel's opinion, but not necessarily to be bound by it.

The minutes of this meeting were published in the *Veterinary Record* of 24th April 1897, and now the rank and file of the profession gave tongue in the correspondence columns. Views ranged from sad resignation at the inevitability of progress, through facetiousness and sentimentality to passionate outrage. The elections to Council were imminent, and it was customary for candidates to write to the *Record* stating their views on current topics and soliciting votes. Mr H. Kidd, a founder member and past secretary to the Royal Counties Veterinary Association, was the only candidate to mention this controversial issue in his election address, saying quite simply "I am in favour of ladies being admitted to the examinations and receiving the Diploma of the RCVS". He was *not* elected, and his assertion provoked an anonymous colleague to an effusion that is worth quoting at length:-

"Sir, Am I dreaming? No!".

He then quoted Kidd's election address and continued:

"Great Scott! What next? Surely an individual who makes use of such astounding language in an appeal for the votes of his *confrères* must be utterly devoid of common sense. When, a short time since, a similar project hailed from America (The land of sensations) it was received with a storm of well deserved scorn and ridicule by the press and sensible people generally, but now that it gains the support of one who has a seat on the governing body of the RCVS right thinking people look aghast at such humbug and foolery, for it is nothing better. Where are the viragos to follow such a calling? Thank goodness in my humble estimation they are few and far between. Certainly there are many callings from which women have been excluded that they can and should competently fill, but that of a veterinary surgeon is out of the question entirely and no true womanly nature would tolerate such an idea. Nor is a woman physically fit or would it be decent for her to castrate, fire, calve, foal, or many other jobs that a busy veterinary surgeon is constantly doing. There is a delicacy over such matters, proper that it should be; I know this from a lifelong experience, having as it were been born a veterinary surgeon, even so among farmers's wives who know the nature of such things, up to now I have never heard of one castrating, foaling or calving; although I will confess that on two solitary occasions, once at a calving and the other at a foaling, I had feminine aid when none other was forthcoming; but must say that it was most reluctantly and modestly rendered. ...If Mr Kidd has been on the Council for eight years it is quite time that the services of such a `dreamer´ were dispensed with..."

He signed himself `A Fellow from the Country´ and the letter appeared in the *Veterinary Record* of 22nd May 1897.

He was supported, in the issue of 5th June, by a more sophisticated but equally passionate diatribe by `W. B. Junior´.

"... The medical schools may open their doors, but let us pray to the gods for strength to keep ours closed. Is it not galling enough to have to meet, and hear of, men in the profession who are not gentlemen without having added to the number of ungentlemanly vets an equal number of `ungentlemanly women´. `Some men can sometimes be gentlemen, but no woman can´ is an apparently absurd remark made by an eminent novelist when speaking of the new woman. There is also to be considered the second and more selfish reason - that of the overcrowding of an already overcrowded profession..."

The correspondence continued for some weeks, the published letters being evenly divided for and against, and the Editor wrote on a number of occasions that `several interesting communications are unavoidably held over´. It is interesting to find that while those in favour of admitting women were all signed, those against were anonymous. At about this time the authorities of Cambridge University declined by a large majority to give degrees to ladies, and this was gleefully reported in the *Veterinary Record* of 12th June as a news item, together with a puerile comment quoted from a Cambridge periodical.

On a more serious note, the learned Counsel's opinion was published in the *Record* of 1st May 1897, as follows:-

"Ladies as Veterinary Surgeons.

A lady student has qualified for her first professional examination, but the Council hesitate to take the step of admitting her. They are supported by the following Counsel's opinion:-

Although the word `student` is applicable to both sexes, I am afraid the intention is manifest everywhere in the Act of qualifying only men. Having regard to this fact, and the fact that in the case of the medical profession it was deemed necessary to pass a special Act, viz., 39 and 40 Vict., C.41, to enable women to become registered practitioners, I think the case is too doubtful to justify the Council to take the important step of admitting women without the authority of a court of law. I should, therefore, advise the council to refuse to admit the lady, and invite her to *mandamus* them. This refusal should be framed in such a way as to raise the point of law and exclude any possibility of discretion."

(Signed `Morton W. Smith`, Temple, 15/4/1897)

This seems to have meant that `Miss Custance` would have to take the initiative herself in taking the RCVS to court to show why she should not be admitted.

According to Mr Thatcher, the College Solicitor, he had some correspondence with Miss Custance's solicitor and invited her to *mandamus* the RCVS in the Queen's Bench Division, offering, at the same time, to make all admissions, so that the only question to be tried was whether lady students had the same right as male students. Miss Custance tried to get such a trial in the Scottish Courts, but Thatcher refused, saying it would be far cheaper and more expeditious to do as he proposed, and that if the proceedings were taken at once there would be time for the lady to come up for the May examinations, assuming her to be successful in her contention.

It is not known why Aleen did not do this, but it may well have been because she was afraid that with the publicity of a law suit in London her real identity might be revealed. This could have damaged, her mother's position at Court, and even if it did not, her mother's disapproval would undoubtedly have made itself felt, backed up by all her aristocratic friends and relations in and around the Court circles. She may also have been hampered by sheer lack of money, and despite Thatcher's protestations about its cheapness she may not have felt able to initiate proceedings on her own account against such a formidable enemy. For whatever reason she did nothing, but an apparent rescue attempt was made by Professor William Williams, Principal of the New Edinburgh College, and his son, Professor Owen Williams, a member of the RCVS Council. These two sued the RCVS and claimed damages from them because they had refused to examine one of their candidates, who had taken the first year's course and was suitably qualified to present herself. This action was brought in the Scottish Courts for the professors' convenience, and although Aleen confessed in later life that she contributed to the expenses of this action she was not officially involved, and could keep completely behind the scenes.

The case was heard at the Court of Sessions, Edinburgh, on Tuesday the 6th June 1897. By a piece of unashamed trickery the RCVS managed to get a ruling that the court had no jurisdiction over it because the RCVS had no domicile in Scotland, and the action was declared null and void. The plaintiffs could have appealed, or they could have brought a fresh action in the English Courts, but they did neither of these things. Aleen had shot her bolt, and she did not again try to gain legal entry into the profession until 1922.

In actual fact the RCVS *were* `domiciled´ in Scotland, because having three of the four veterinary colleges in Scotland they had always had an office there with their own headed notepaper. Thatcher admitted that had a sheet of this been produced in court they would have lost the case and been forced to defend the action on its merits. It is interesting to note that most commentators seemed to assume that if the case had been fairly debated in court the pro-feminists would have won, but that most of the Council viewed this prospect with inarticulate horror. It was not till the meeting of 13th January 1898 that they felt the danger of further legal action had receded sufficiently for them to discuss it. While congratulating themselves on their lucky escape they spent an inordinate amount of time trying to find a way of continuing to use their Scottish office and having its address on their notepaper without laying themselves open to a charge of being domiciled in Scotland. They never did succeed in solving this problem, but as the case was not reopened it did not matter.

In her letter to the *Record* of 1934 Miss Cust says she herself also took Counsel's opinion. Being a private person she had to pay fifteen guineas - which she could ill afford - instead of the RCVS standing Counsel's two, and she was told that although she was probably in the right she would be unwise to proceed unless her purse was `very deep´ as her adversaries would fight it all the way to the House of Lords, where so many of her censorious relatives were ensconced. So she drew in her horns and studied hard, if unofficially. In suing for `loss of fees´ Professor Williams implied that she would not continue her studies and would leave the College forthwith, but she stayed on for the remaining three years to complete the full course of training. She did not again present herself for any of the RCVS examinations, but she was evidently a very good student as in her first year she gained the gold medal for zoology. Moreover, old Andrew Spreull, a highly respected practitioner in Dundee, allowed Aleen to `see practice´ (i.e. go as a pupil) with him during one of her vacations, and according to his grandson, he alleged that Aleen was the best student he had ever had. One of his own sons was in Aleen's class in Edinburgh, and it seems they were neck and neck in winning the medals awarded in the first year. After this first year, however, Aleen's name does not appear in any of the awards, so perhaps she was deemed ineligible for them. It would be interesting to know if they charged her full fees for those last three years. They would have been justified in doing so, as veterinary teaching is notoriously expensive because of the need to dissect the larger domestic animals, and because of the detailed clinical tuition; but they may have made some reduction for her as she was not allowed to sit the examinations.

While studying in Edinburgh she often visited the Widdringtons at Newton Hall, and she may have spent much of her vacations there. The wild countryside, spacious gardens, and above all the stables, must have been a welcome change from her spartan conditions in Edinburgh. Even more important was the friendship and moral support they gave her, approving and applauding her studies and successes. Her own family were scandalized by her behaviour and would have nothing more to do with her. By this time her brother Charles was equerry to the Queen's grandson, who was later to become George Vth. They saw much less of Charles at Newton Hall because, as one of Fitz's grandsons put it, `he had become a courtier´.

In 1900 Aleen left College with a testimonial from Principal Williams, certifying that she had attended the full course and proved herself competent in all subjects. On his recommendation she had obtained a post as assistant to William Byrne, MRCVS, of Roscommon in Ireland, and thus began her career in general practice.

Probably the die-hards on the RCVS Council hoped she would either die or get married within a few years, either of these fates being lethal to most careers for women, but to their subsequent discomfort she avoided both.

CHAPTER III

In Practice

"Work apace, apace, apace,
Honest labour bears a lovely face"

Thomas Dekker - `Sweet Content'

William Augustine Byrne was born in Roscommon in 1864. His parents died when he was a child, and he and his two brothers were brought up by various relatives, first in Dublin and later in Ballydooly. He had an unusually broad education, first taking a course in agriculture at Glasnevin, and then studying classics with a private tutor in Castlerea and Brandon. From there he went to the Royal Veterinary College, London, where he is said to have taken the four years course in only three years, presumably because of his agricultural degree. He obtained his MRCVS in May 1889 at the age of twenty-five, staying on at the Royal Veterinary College for a further year as House Surgeon and Demonstrator in Anatomy.

One of his uncles was a millionaire, who had made his money in America, and then died, leaving his nephew a castle in Athleague and enough money to set him up comfortably in practice in the year 1890. `Castlestrange' is now a picturesque ivy clad ruin, but in those days Byrne lived there and practised from there until his death in 1910.

He was a brilliant young man, handsome and witty, and became very popular with colleagues and clients. It is said that he was a fine poet, although none of his work has survived. He was certainly very eloquent, with a command of language that could be charming or devastatingly sarcastic as he chose. He was very much a ladies man - some say something of a libertine who had fathered several illegitimate children - but he remained a good Catholic and so popular that any scandalous stories could be put down to envy or malice. The ink was scarce dry on his Diploma before he wrote an exuberant letter to the *Veterinary Record* complaining bitterly because the students were kept waiting an unnecessarily long time for their examination results.

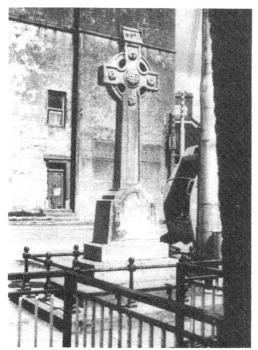

William Byrne's monument, Roscommon

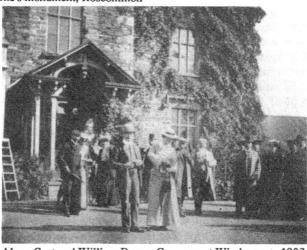

Aleen Cust and William Byrne, Congress at Windermere, 1903

26

Once back in Roscommon he threw himself into local activities with boundless energy. From earliest boyhood he had been a fervent nationalist, and for a number of years he was president of the Athleague branch of the United Irishmen's league. He was also secretary of the Roscommon Harrier Hunt, and he once boasted that the Roscommon Staghounds were the fastest pack of hounds in Ireland.

He brought the same enthusiasm and energy into veterinary politics, and in 1897 was a founder member of the Irish Central Veterinary Society. In October of that year, a few months after the lawsuit in Edinburgh over Aleen's candidature, he read a paper to the Society on `Veterinary Ethics´, which contained the following paragraph:-

> `Man's treatment of woman is one of the most absorbing and difficult ethical questions of today, as it has been for all time. I cannot leave the question of veterinary ethics without adverting to the discussion which has arisen within our ranks as to the admission of women to the veterinary profession. George Meredith is the only novelist I know of, whom women admit knows their sex. I never knew anyone else who knew them. But I think we can all admit this knowledge, that, though the difficulties may seem insuperable, lovely women " get there in the end". Women will, of course, be admitted to the veterinary profession. If there is a majority of mysogynous old bachelors and henpecked husbands on the Council their admission may be delayed, but it will come. Why any woman who loves a horse or dog - or, as many of them do, all dumb things - will not be allowed to acquire a knowledge of their diseases, is a thing I cannot understand. Nor can I comprehend the mental attitude of those who insist that there is no work for a woman veterinary surgeon except castration and obstetrics.´

All this amused his audience very much, and there were several facetious comments and advice to the handsome young bachelor, but nobody else seemed to be considering the problem seriously. Nevertheless there is a personal tone in his remarks which suggests that he may have already met Aleen Cust. Principal Williams was extremely keen that his students should `see practice´ as much as possible during their college days. This meant staying in a veterinary surgeon's household, or very near it, and assisting him at his work and learning from him. The rules about `unqualified assistants´ - who were strictly discouraged because of the danger of them subsequently setting up as `quacks` - were always waived for *bona fide* students, and the unofficial tuition and experience gained in this way was reckoned almost as important as the college lectures. Aleen may have chosen to see practice in Ireland, partly because she liked the country and its people, but also because she would be less likely to be recognised there than in rural England, where she had probably been hunting in every county from the Midlands to Northumberland. Examinations at the New Edinburgh College were always held in May to give the studens a maximum time to see practice before the next session started in October. Aleen could have seen practice for several months, even if she had waited for the outcome of the lawsuit in June, or she may have felt it wise to be out of Edinburgh at the time of the trial and gone off as soon as she knew that she could not take the examination in May. While it is unlikely that they would place her with a young unmarried practitioner, Byrne could well have been introduced to her by a colleague, or perhaps met her in the hunting field if she had been allowed time off for such pursuits.

In 1900 the Dublin Veterinary College was founded, and the National Veterinary Association (the old name for the present British Veterinary Association) held its Annual Congress in Dublin. This Congress is mainly scientific, but is also an important occasion socially. It lasts about a week and veterinary surgeons are encouraged to bring their wives and children and make it a family holiday. It falls to the local veterinary association to help organise the scientific programme and to be almost wholly responsible for the social side. This includes a `ladies` programme to keep the wives and sweethearts pleasurably occupied while their menfolk attend the scientific sessions, and there are also joint functions when the whole company goes off to excursions, garden parties, civic receptions, and so on, culminating in the annual banquet. This is a heavy responsibility for the local association, and the president and other officers are in the position of hosts to the Congress.

At the Annual General Meeting of the Irish Central Veterinary Society in July 1899 there was much deliberation about the election of the president for the following year. As the chairman, Mr E. C. Winter, said: `This year is an especially important one for the Irish veterinary surgeons and it is essential that we should be careful to put the right man in the right place.` That the choice for president eventually fell on young Mr Byrne was a great compliment to him, and he was very sensible of the honour. In May of 1900 he and Mr Winter were also nominated for the Council of the RCVS. The inauguration of the Dublin College made it highly desirable to have some Irish representatives on the Council, and both men were elected for a term of four years.

28

These responsibilities involved William Byrne in a lot of extra work, and he decided he needed an assistant to help him in his practice and to take full charge when he had to be away on business. To the astonishment of his colleagues and friends the new assistant was a woman - Aleen Cust. She came on the strong recommendation of Principal Williams, who explained that she was fully trained, although the refusal of the RCVS to admit her to their examinations meant that she had no Diploma, was not on the Register, and must never be called a veterinary surgeon in public. This odd situation would have daunted a lesser man and outraged a conventional circle of English County families, but with the Irish genius for practicalities - it worked! Aleen was competent enough to satisfy her employer, and her mixture of aristocratic finesse and an earthy understanding of people and animals charmed the whole rural community. All, that is, except the Roman Catholic clergy. To them she was an anomaly that ought not to have happened. William Byrne told the priest that she was engaged by correspondence and he had no idea she was a woman until she arrived, and he had then found her lodgings in Athleague. This may have been a polite fiction to satisfy the priest of the propriety of the arrangements, or it may have been true, and the partnership entirely professional.

The relationship between these two strong personalities is interesting and ambiguous. They worked together for some years, some say lived together as man and wife, although in 1905 she was living at Ballygar, some miles to the South. In 1900 she was thirty-two and he thirty-six, and both were unattached and physically attractive. Yet she was too much a woman of the world to be easily swept off her feet, even by Willie Byrne, and he too was neither naive nor inexperienced. In a small rural community it was inevitable that rumours should arise, but the high regard that Irish veterinary surgeons seem to have had for Miss Cust suggests that if she and Byrne were lovers they were very discreet about it. There is a tale - at least third hand, and unconfirmed - of a violent quarrel between them. Aleen had borrowed one of his favourite horses, and ridden it so hard that it was in a state of collapse and had to be shot. William told her to get off his premises and said that if she did not he would shoot her too. Evidently she went, but by this time she seems to have been more or less independent, and her reputation with the farmers was such that she could survive without him, despite her legal disabilities. However, he seems to have continued to befriend her, recommending her for a post with the Galway County Council in 1905, and discreetly introducing her as `a visitor´ at various veterinary meetings and conferences. Without his help she could never have

29

become accepted so quickly by her male colleagues, in spite of her professional competence.

If Aleen might have been tempted to form a liaison that would advance her career she was soon to be tempted more severely by an affair which could have ruined it. Bertram, the son of her beloved guardian Major `Fitz `Widdrington, in whose home she had spent so many happy days, was now a tall handsome young Army officer; and in the summer of 1904 he was home on leave from India. Aleen seems to have left Bryne's employment by then and managed to spend quite a lot of time in Northumberland, and also went on holiday with the Widdringtons to Scotland. Bertram wanted her to marry him, and eventually she agreed. His parents were somewhat dismayed, as they understood only too well Aleen's obsession with veterinary work, and although she was very much in love, they could not see her giving up her work to become a conventional Army wife. As Bertram himself ruefully commented, he knew Aleen would not be tolerated in India by `the Regiment' who believed in `feminine women'. He was two years younger than Aleen, and so infatuated with her that he contemplated giving up his Army career in order to accommodate her. They discussed the possibility of living at Low Hall, near Newton Hall where his parents lived, so that Aleen might set up in practice there, at least until child-bearing overtook her. However, after he went back to India the engagement was apparently broken off by correspondence. Aleen had a strong sense of fair play, and I suspect that on sober consideration she would have been as horrified at Bertram giving up his career as at a similar sacrifice of her own. So she went back to Ireland, and the lonely struggles of her legal balancing act, and a few years later Bertram married someone more suitable.

How much was Aleen affected by this? One cannot say, but she never forgot Bertram. For the rest of her days she seems to have dealt with the men around her with unfailing tact and friendliness, but with a complete evasion of overt entanglement. For a successful career woman a romantic attachment to someone in another continent is as good a fireguard as any against emotional involvement nearer home, so perhaps Bertram helped her more than he knew.

For those familiar with the hectic pace of agricultural veterinary practice, as described by James Herriot, it must be pointed out that things were somewhat different in Ireland in the early part of the twentieth century. Professor H. A. Woodruff, who was at one time editor of the independent weekly publication *Veterinary News*, gave `Some Holiday

Impressions of Irish Practice´ in an editorial of 24th September 1910, from which are quoted the following extracts:-

`The first thing one notices is the great respect, nay, almost veneration, that all and sundry have for "the docther" provided, of course, that he is a sportsman. In England it is possible for a veterinary surgeon to succeed whilst having little of the sportsman about him, but such a thing is almost impossible in Ireland. The motor car - ubiquitous in England - is much less common in Ireland, and although the state of the roads in many parts may be partly answerable yet the love of the horse is so intimately a part of the Irishman's constitution that one cannot conceive of much decay in horse practice there. Among any collection of Irishmen the main topics of conversation are usually hunting, racing, horse fairs, or sport, and in the world of sport the Irishman is surely a prince. This it is that gives the Irish veterinary practitioner his unique position, for he is looked upon as an authority on these matters, and let him see to it that he fails not here. Examinations for soundness form a large part of his work, and may be as severe a test of the veterinary surgeon as of the horse, for the Irish farmer client will often deliberately suppress vital information to see "will the docther find it out". Every horseman loves a good deal; he likes good looks and quality, but more still he must have a good performer. He will pay comparatively little attention to those unfortunate little bony excrescences to which horses are heirs, provided the animal can gallop and "lep" and the "pipes are all right". Testing the wind of a horse is a serious business in Ireland. A very pleasing feature is the respect paid to advice and the little concern for medicine. It is much easier to obtain a reasonable fee for advice in Ireland than in England, and there is in consequence little need for the supply of pills, lotions, drenches and powders which pay the rent in some practices nearer home. The people do not appear to have such boundless faith in medicine that many in England appear to have, and as a result empiricism is much less prevalent in Ireland. Many practitioners appear to dispense no medicines but to prescribe what is necessary and allow the chemist to supply it.

There is much good fellowship and *camaraderie* among practitioners in Ireland. They are often spaced far apart, and a man may have no opposition whatever in a whole county. This being so it is perhaps the more remarkable in what light-hearted

31

fashion "the docther" will leave his practice for a day or more while he goes racing, or to a fair or show. The Dublin Horse Show week must indeed be a bad week for any unfortunate animal taken sick in the country districts, for the profession is in Dublin almost to a man.

The work of the Department of Agriculture and Technical Instruction is very important, and one had only to visit the south and west to see how beneficent and multiform are the Department's activities. It has throughout made much use of the veterinary practitioners, and as a consequence they are keen and loyal servants, and by allowing local problems to be dealt with by the man on the spot many difficulties have been overcome.

There is a sense of unity and combination among veterinary surgeons in Ireland for the purpose of defending and securing their rights and privileges, for example they have obtained freedom from jury service, and the profession in Ireland supplies an object lesson in the value of amalgamation and combination.´

Such a world seems almost to have been designed specially to accommodate Aleen Cust. Her passion for horses and her already extensive knowledge of them were a prime qualification, while her quick brain had absorbed all the science and art that the four years training at Edinburgh could give her. The meticulous attention to detail that marked all she did would ensure that it was all put to good use. Add a warm heart, and a personal charm worthy of the Irish themselves, and she could hardly go wrong.

She arrived at Willie Byrne's practice in May 1900, and the first few months would have been spent visiting cases with him and being introduced to all his more important clients. In August the National Veterinary Congress was held in Dublin, and as president of the local Veterinary Association Byrne was wholly preoccupied by it. Aleen took no part in this Congress, and was presumably left holding the fort - the first major test of her ability. A veterinary surgeon rarely gets an assistant until he has for some time been struggling with more work than he can handle. There is always an awkward period when clients may resent being fobbed off with a younger and less experienced person. Then, gradually, the position changes until that piquant moment when clients begin to `ask for´ the new assistant. A sensible practitioner accepts this with relief, though he would hardly be human if he did not sometimes feel a twinge of surprise or even downright jealousy. When the Congress was over and Willie back in harness he found that the clients had already taken Aleen to their hearts, and her position was assured.

The next few years were probably among the happiest in her life. She was doing work she loved, and becoming increasingly good at it, and she was accepted and appreciated by all around her. She seems to have become independent of Willie Byrne quite soon, but she lived only a few miles away and they remained good friends. As her reputation grew he gradually introduced her to the local Veterinary Association, and although she took no part in the formal discussions, her presence was accepted and her professional ability respected.

She was very conscious of her debt of gratitude to Principal William Williams of the New Edinburgh Veterinary College for procuring her this situation, and soon after her arrival in Ireland the following letter appeared in the *North British Agriculturalist*, and was reproduced in the *Veterinary Record* of 23rd June 1900, and in other veterinary periodicals:-

"Dear Professor Williams,

Remembering the many kindnesses which I have received from you, and also the fact that to you I owe the present position which I now occupy, I would like in some way to express my gratitude. Therefore, if you will kindly allow me, I will give a prize of £25 annually for the next four years, to be competed for by students of the New Veterinary College, Edinburgh. I would suggest that the prize should be given to the student who obtains the highest aggregate number of marks in his A, B, C and D examinations of the Royal College of Veterinary Surgeons; also that the student must have been regular in his attendance and of good behaviour during the time he has attended the New Veterinary College.

The first prize to be awarded after the examination in 1901. And I may say that, should I still be living in the land of prosperity at the expiration of the four years, and the giving of the prizes prove to be the success which I sincerely hope they will be, I shall do my best to consider giving the prize annually.

If there is any other scheme that you think would be more advantageous to the student or the welfare of the profession, I shall be very pleased to hear from you on the subject.

In giving these prizes I wish to be "anonymous" - with every good wish, believe me, ever yours faithfully,

`An old student´."

This was almost certainly from Aleen. It is most unlikely that any other `Old Student´ would do such a thing, and something in the style, and the meticulous, finicking detail resembles the many and complicated provisions of the Will she made in later life. The prize was duly given, but it seems to have stopped after 1903. Principal Williams died in the autumn of 1900, and she may have terminated the arrangement after discussion with his son, Professor Owen Williams, who succeeded his father as Principal, and who was present at the 1903 National Veterinary Congress at Windermere. This Congress, held in September 1903, was highly successful, and an editorial in the *Veterinary Record* says it was `Perhaps the most fully representative that the Association has held.´ William Byrne was there, and for the first time Aleen Cust's name appears in the list of `visitors.´

In the *Veterinary Record* of 10th October 1903, there are several photographs, including one of Aleen and William captioned `The lady v.s. and the Irish Poet´. The photographs were taken by Mr H. J. Dawes, the secretary of the Midland Counties Veterinary Association, who practised in West Bromwich. The designation `v.s.´ is sailing rather close to the wind, and could well have been disapproved by the old guard of the RCVS Council, but as no names were mentioned, it got by. It was evidently unposed, and shows Aleen, very tall, with a long full skirt and broad-brimmed hat, rummaging in her handbag, while William looks on impassively.

At the Congress banquet William replied to the toast of `The Ladies´ in what was evidently an extremely witty speech, but nobody seems to have been in a fit condition to report it in detail, so as with his poems, we have only the effect on others by which to judge it. In those days women did not seem to have spoken in public at such gatherings, and a man was always deputed to answer the toast for them.

In May 1904 Byrne's term of office on the RCVS Council ended. He had faithfully attended nearly all the Council meetings, despite the difficulty and expense of travelling to London, and he was duly nominated for re-election, but he did not get in. Quite possibly he was too outspoken for them. His youth, his sarcastic wit, and his contempt for the hair-splitting and in-fighting that undoubtedly went on at Council meetings may well have scandalized the more senior members, and he lost the election by a wide margin. Mr Gooch, of the Lincolnshire Veterinary Association, deplored this and greatly lamented his departure, and some of Byrne's fellow countrymen felt the same, but they could do nothing. If all the Irish members had voted for Byrne he would probably have got in, so their allegiance must have wavered. The Council members were violently agitated by Principal Owen Williams' decision to move the New Edinburgh Veterinary College to Liverpool, making it part of Liverpool University. McFadyean saw this as a possible threat to the Council's control of their examinations for entry into the profession, and this issue dominated all their debates. Byrne does not seem to have associated himself with this hue and cry, and it was those that did who were elected, McFadyean himself topping the poll.

Byrne may have been quite glad to shed some of his responsibilities, however, as that summer the National Veterinary Congress was again to be in Dublin and he would play a prominent part in it. Aleen attended this Congress as a visitor, and although she does not seem to figure recognisably in the official photographs she evidently took many photographs herself, and this is acknowledged in several of those published in the *Veterinary Record*. An editorial of the issue of 27th August also records that Professor Mettam, Principal of the Dublin College, gave a demonstration with lantern and screen of a very fine collection of microphotographs of pathological subjects. Evidently the `visitors´ were allowed in on this, for the Editor remarks `None of the ladies were ill and one was delighted´ which may well have referred to Aleen. She undoubtedly used these occasions to ingratiate herself with her male colleagues, gradually enlarging the circle of those who knew her and accepted her as one of themselves.

1905 was a busy and significant year for Aleen. William Byrne went to London for several months to take a post-graduate course run by Professor McFadyean, now principal of the Royal Veterinary College, London. McFadyean was then at the height of his powers. He had a degree in human medicine as well as his veterinary qualification, and he was among the first veterinary surgeons to do serious research into animal diseases, using to the full the comparatively young sciences of bacteriology and pathology. He was also an excellent teacher, and the powerfully outspoken editor of the *Journal of Comparative Pathology*. It is typical of Byrne's professional acumen and scholarly disposition that he sought to reinforce his considerable clinical experience and expertise by taking such a course and getting up to date in scientific theory.

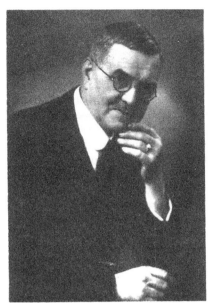

Sir Frederick Hobday, FRCVS

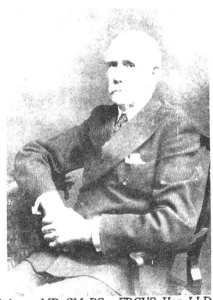

Sir John McFadyean, MB, CM, BSc., FRCVS, Hon. LLD
(Aberdeen), FRS (Edinburgh)

He had engaged a locum tenens to look after his practice, but the unfortunate man suffered a stroke soon after Byrne's departure and became a permanent invalid. This must have thrown considerably more work on Aleen, who was Byrne's nearest neighbouring practitioner. McFadyean's course was a great success, and in March 1905 his class of fifteen post-graduate students gave a dinner in his honour.

The National Veterinary Congress was at Buxton that year and although Byrne did not go, Aleen did, and again she took some photographs which were published, with suitable acknowledgment, in the *Veterinary Record*. Then, in September 1905, Aleen went to the 8th International Veterinary Congress at Budapest. Only six British people were present at this function - a fact regretted in editorial comment. Aleen attended `privately´ and was no doubt a conspicuous ornament to the meagre British contingent, especially as she spoke both French and German fluently. After the Congress she went with the delegates on the post-congress tour to the Royal Estates and horse-breeding establishments of the Archduke's farm in Hungary. She took some very good photographs here also, and some of these were published in the *Veterinary Record* and the *Veterinary Journal*. Moreover, Professor Hobday, who was present as a delegate from the Central Veterinary Society of London, when he reported back to them with an account of the Budapest Congress used slides made from some of Aleen's photographs. The English party included McFadyean and his son-in-law Stewart Stockman. Both these eminent veterinary surgeons were implacably opposed to the entry of women into the profession, and one can only speculate on their reactions to Aleen's presence, but Professor Hobday became her friend for life.

But Aleen's greatest gain from her presence at Budapest came in February 1906 when she was invited to read a paper to the Irish Central Veterinary Association. She chose her subject skilfully - `A trip to the Imperial Horse-breeding Studs and Large Herds of Hungary and Serbia´, and it was illustrated by her own lantern slides. Nobody could attack her for presuming to speak on a strictly veterinary subject, yet it was one to get most Irish veterinary surgeons consumed with interest, and it permitted her to display her knowledge of horses and everything about them in a way that proclaimed her every inch a veterinary surgeon. There was a good discussion, and many tributes to the essayist for her `instructive and graphic lecture´. The meetings of the Irish Central were regularly reported in the *Veterinary Record*, but not a word was printed about this meeting. Whether the secretary omitted to send it in, or whether he sent it in and it was ceremonially burnt at the Editorial Office of the National Veterinary Association we shall never know, but the meeting was reported at length in the *Irish Times*, and this report was quoted in full by the lively little *Veterinary News*, whose editor specialised in differing from the official *Veterinary Record* whenever he thought fit.

CHAPTER IV

The Controversial Inspector

"It's hundreds are your friends, my daughter,
It's thousands are your foe"

Ballad of Lord Thomas and Fair Elenor - Anon.

So far Aleen was quietly consolidating her position with the insidious persistence of a stray cat getting inside the kitchen, but in the months that followed she made a more positive bid for official recognition. There was a vacancy under the Galway County Council for a Veterinary Inspector to administer the official Acts and orders concerning the diseases of animals. It was a part-time post, and it was the custom to employ a local practitioner who could combine the duties with his private practice. Aleen was one of three who applied for the post, the other two being male and on the Register of Veterinary Surgeons. Nevertheless, the Galway County Council selected Aleen, who was now well known in the area, as the most suitable candidate.

This appointment set off a storm in the Royal College of Veterinary Surgeon's Council which reverberated all round the profession and the Department of Agriculture for months. It is evident from the local newspaper account of the meeting of the Galway County Council that they were fully aware of Miss Cust's anomalous position, but nevertheless regarded her as the most suitable candidate, and she was chosen by a vote of 14 to 10. A week later this was reported in the *Veterinary Record* of 11th November 1905. A full column of the editorial is devoted to it, and the facts are fairly ventilated. The following extracts are quoted:-

> "The Galway County Council has appointed a person who is not a MRCVS but a lady. This sort of action `agin the Government´ could take place nowhere except in Ireland, but even there must be sharply looked after by the Corporate Body, who are threatened with a breach of their privileges... We do not dispute Miss Cust's intelligence or acquirements for the post, but as she

39

does not possess the licence to practice granted by the diploma of the RCVS her appointment is obviously a trespass upon their domain."

They had to admit one loophole, however, by which Ireland was again considered to be exceptional, this time officially:-

"The Diseases of Animals Act requires each local authority to appoint at least one Veterinary Inspector", and a `Veterinary Inspector´ is defined as a Member of the RCVS. Unfortunately the Act (Section 69) says that "The provisions of this Act requiring local authorities to keep appointed Veterinary Inspectors shall not extend to Ireland" but it also provides that the Lord Lieutenant may make such orders in Council as to him seem fit "for defining the qualifications and powers of inspectors".

The editorial therefore asserted that the Department of Agriculture had full powers `to veto improper appointments´ and should reject this one. It ended with the quaintly ambiguous statement:-

"It would be strange indeed if we were to be undone by the appointment of a lady who has no diploma, simply because she is a lady. No man, even in Galway, could have driven through our Act, but if once the breach is made men without diplomas will follow."

The protestations continued in the editorial of the week following. Describing the member of the Galway County Council who proposed Miss Cust's appointment as `an aggressive person´ it continued that:-

"... he made the mysterious remark `If the question of qualification is going to be raised now I might feel compelled to adopt a course which I do not like to take.´ Whether this meant that he could withdraw his proposal, or anything more dreadful, we cannot say, but he later declared that `Miss Cust had the highest legal opinion that the RCVS were wrong in not admitting her a member´.

Possibly all this was `bluff´ but it may mean more. It may mean the prelude to another action against the RCVS with the accompanying costs.

> There is only one excuse for the Galway County Council, viz.,
> that they looked upon Miss Cust as a martyr to the narrow
> prejudices of the veterinary profession, and that they accepted the
> statements of the writers of her testimonials as to fitness."

The editorial then quoted a list of five veterinary surgeons, headed by
Professor Owen Williams, now principal of the `New´ Edinburgh
Veterinary College which had been moved to Liverpool, and admonished
them that:

> "We think they are ill advised to allow their personal feelings to
> guide them in what might have been a severe blow to their
> profession."

This may at first sight look like an incredibly violent storm in a very
small teacup, but the nub of the matter is revealed in that pathetic
sentence about an action with accompanying costs. In 1897 when the
RCVS had bulldozed their way through a lawsuit which, however
irrationally, slammed the door of their examination rooms in Miss Cust's
face, she was an unknown and impoverished student and they were a
very powerful body of men. Now Miss Cust was an established and
wealthy practitioner, recognised by eminent Irish veterinary surgeons as
their equal in training, competence and integrity. And the RCVS? It was
heading down a slippery slope to bankruptcy. The fees of students no
longer covered the expense of examining them, and their governing Act
of Parliament did not empower the Council to raise money by any other
means. Had the profession been discreet and united they could probably
have got a new Bill through Parliament as an agreed measure, which
would have given them the power to charge a modest annual fee to any
person wishing to remain on the Register. This arrangement is in force
today for the RCVS and most other professional bodies. But a number of
prominent veterinary surgeons had refused to sanction this annual levy
on those already qualified, and others raised conditions about the
payment, declaring that if the RCVS had a new Act of Parliament it
should insist on a clause preventing `quackery´ - that is, the practising of
veterinary surgery and medicine by unqualified people. This incurred
the wrath of the farming community, many of whom regularly employed
unqualified men for much things as the gelding of young male pigs,
lambs and calves. Such men were often highly respected members of the
rural community, specialising in that simple operation which they did
quite adequately and for a much smaller fee than that of a veterinary

41

surgeon. The rural landowners were a powerful force, and although the offending clause was hastily dropped from the draft of the Bill they remained deeply suspicious, and could completely prevent it going through as an agreed measure.

Had the profession been united a short debate might have sufficed to allay the farmers' fears and give the RCVS the funds it needed, but the argumentative Mr Dollar was on the Council and was able to muster all the forces of greed and conservatism which lurk beneath the skin of men whose living depends on business acumen, although they aspire to be regarded as a learned profession. It did not matter that a referendum of the profession showed a sound majority in favour of the annual fee. The minority was vociferous and articulate, and included men of great reputation and seniority. Every year the treasurer warned of the consequences, and every year more and more of their capital had to be sold at a loss to pay current expenses. The RCVS was becoming increasingly powerless and could not afford to finance lawsuits for any but the most blatant trespasses against it. The case for admitting women to the profession was now being backed by many of the members of Ireland, and by several professors, especially of the Liverpool School, which was now situated within Liverpool University, where women had long been admitted to most of the other faculties.

Aleen did not need actually to bring an action against the RCVS. Her discreetly leaked hints to the Galway County Council were quite enough to spread panic throughout the RCVS Council. They determined to oppose her appointment by every means in their power, but needed to do it with a minimum of publicity, to avoid the astonishment and derision of the intelligentsia outside the British profession. For women could now train as veterinary surgeons in France, Russia, America and Australia, so why not in Britain?

Not all the Irish approved of Aleen. A paragraph reprinted in the *Veterinary Record* from the *Ballinasloe Western News* reads:-

> `The County Council have made an appointment in the horse and brute kingdom which appears to us at least disgusting, if not absolutely indecent! Of the many callings embraced by women, that of judging and doctoring horses appears to us the most unsuitable and repulsive. We can understand women educating themselves to tend women - but horses! heavens!´

Moreover the Irish Veterinary Medical Association, the senior of the two veterinary associations in Ireland, wrote to the Department of

Agriculture approving of their refusal to sanction the appointment and urging them to stand firm. The independent *Veterinary News* also thought that this appointment was too much, and said that Miss Cust had been put in a ridiculous position.

The monthly *Veterinary Journal*, however, of November 1905, in a very balanced and fair editorial, set out the history of Miss Cust's career and explained her suitability for the post. This was followed up in the December issue by a letter, almost certainly from William Byrne, although his surname is mis-spelt, in which he defended Miss Cust and said the sensible way out of the dilemma was for the RCVS to pass a resolution in Council granting her the diploma *honoris causa*, so that she could be placed on the Register forthwith. This suggestion must have sent some councillors' blood pressure dangerously high, but the Department had by this time definitely forbidden the appointment, and insisted that the post be readvertised.

This was done, but the Galway County Council still maintained that they could find no other suitable candidate. Many years later, in one of Miss Cust's obituaries, it was stated that the local Irish veterinary surgeons deliberately boycotted this advertisement out of `gallantry´. It is probably nearer the truth to say that since one of the conditions of the appointment was that the holder should live in the district, nobody wanted to put his professional plate up in the area of such a successful practitioner as Miss Cust. After their meeting in May 1906 the Galway County Council therefore reappointed Miss Cust. This drew forth in the correspondence columns of the *Veterinary Record* an anonymous letter which contained the following:-

> "I don't see the use of sending our boys to College at very big expense when we can make our daughters `v.s.´ and veterinary inspectors without any cost. I would like the names of the eminent MRCVS who gave this lady all the credentials she is able to produce.
>
> I am, Sir, Yours truly,
> Irish Country Practitioner."

As the names had been published in full in the *Veterinary Record* a few months previously, he was evidently not a very retentive reader.

Meanwhile the Veterinary Medical Association of Ireland's Council decided to publish the whole of their correspondence with the Irish Department of Agriculture on this vexed question. In response to their agitation they had been given a copy of the Department's letter to the Galway Council Council of 6th June 1906, which stated that:-

> "In view of the circumstances ... the department are prepared to acquiesce in the appointment, as a provisional arrangement, ... of Miss Cust as an Inspector - not a Veterinary Inspector - under the Diseases of Animals Act ... It should be clearly understood that as Miss Cust is not a duly qualified veterinary surgeon she has no claim to the title of a Veterinary Inspector. Her proper designation will be that of 'Inspector'.

> I am, Sir, your obedient servant etc., etc."

Thus was honour satisfied, and the 'provisional arrangement' continued until 1915, when Miss Cust left Ireland. As one unrepentant councillor put it at the next Council meeting, when they contemplated defying the Department of Agriculture over something else, "They refused to sanction her, but we have her all the same as a veterinary surgeon."

Despite the reticence of the RCVS, the subject of the entry of women into the profession, and in particular the position of Aleen Cust, had come into the open because of the Galway appointment, and many people began to express their opinions about it. Professor George Wooldridge, then at the Dublin Veterinary College, opening the discussion on reforms of the examination system at a meeting of the Veterinary Medical Association of Ireland, quoted a certain eminent but un-named veterinary surgeon as calling the opponents of Miss Cust 'old fogies' and another as saying he recognised Miss Cust as 'a member of my profession'. While Professor Wooldridge was careful to dissociate himself from such heresies, their open proclamation meant that they were worth serious consideration. In August 1907, at another meeting of the same Association, two members openly condemned the RCVS Council's attitude to Miss Cust and said they should be ashamed of themselves, while a third thought the admission of women should be incorporated in the proposed new Veterinary Surgeons' Bill. Wallis Hoare, the essayist of the evening, deplored this digression and said he did not think it would be very pleasant to have ladies in the profession, having regard to their various whims and vagaries, and another senior member backed him up, but the chairman did his best to damp down and curtail this discussion. At a meeting of the Scottish Metropolitan Veterinary Association, a Mr

Cameron of Berwick-on-Tweed also wished to see sex discrimination abolished in the new Veterinary Surgeons' Bill.

In October 1907 Aleen was among the honorary veterinary surgeons for the local Agricultural show, and the *Irish Times* in reporting this designated her as `Miss Cust, MRCVS´. The Irish VMA protested about this, but were told that a newspaper report was `not legal evidence´ and they had no grounds for action.

In November 1907, under the heading `Facts v. Fiction´ the *Veterinary Record* printed without further comment an article about Miss Cust which was a tissue of lies with a few half-truths scattered among them. It implied that the `Aristocratic lady from England´ was a failed student in both Scotland and England who had obtained the Galway appointment because she was a relation of Mr George Wyndham, an ex-Chief Secretary. Whether Aleen was really related to this gentleman is not known, but nearly all her relations had cut Aleen out of their acquaintance because of her espousal of the veterinary profession, and any perusal of the minutes of the Galway County Council's meetings on the subject would have established the true facts. The writer of the article could only have been actuated by malice, and in reprinting it the *Veterinary Record* was also guilty, as those unacquainted with Miss Cust's history could well have been prejudiced against her by this article.

However, Aleen continued to prosper in spite of these calumnies, and in April 1909 there was advertised in the *Veterinary Record* `The Cust Rope Release Hobbles´, manufactured by the well-known Instrument firm of Arnold and Sons, with a diagram and description. Messrs Arnold and Sons could find no record of this in their archives, but said it looked like an improved version of another pattern of horse hobbles which appeared in earlier catalogues. Such hobbles were used to cast horses, that is to throw them to the ground - a highly skilled operation - so that they could be secured lying on one side in preparation for administering an anaesthetic and performing surgery. These particular hobbles were light in weight, simple and inexpensive, and could be adapted for use on any size of animal from a donkey to a heavy draught horse.

Meanwhile William Byrne had been very active in the Irish Central Veterinary Society in proposing amending legislation on tuberculosis in cattle. However, he was beginning to slow down a little, and his attendances became less regular. At a meeting on the 3rd October 1909, he opened the discussion on a clinical paper by his old friend E. C. Winter. He began rather strangely, for him, saying he had a very vivid recollection of the seemingly recent day when he had to apologise for his youth and inexperience. Looking amongst the friends assembled at the meeting he realised with sorrow that twenty years hard work had whitened the flowers of the grave upon his head, and that he was a patriarch among them. Age imposed on him the duty of opening the discussion, but it also gave him the privilege of delegating the task of discussing pathological novelties to the new recruits to their ranks, whom he was glad to notice present. He then went on to discuss chylous ascites in his usual forthright way, and to congratulate the essayist. Byrne was only in his mid-forties, and whether he spoke in jest or earnest, it was uncharacteristic of him. Was it some presentiment, or did he know that he was doomed? As a pathologist he may have already been aware that the small lump in his neck was an early sarcoma. This was the last veterinary meeting he attended. On the 21st October he took the train to Dublin to attend a dinner in honour of Sir Charles Cameron, the Medical Officer of Health for Dublin, who had proved a great friend to the veterinary profession. Willie Byrne never reached that dinner. He was taken ill on the train and had to return home at once to Athleague. He underwent an operation, but his friends were given the impression that it was a minor affair of small consequence, and it came as a great shock to most of them when he died on Sunday the 17th April 1910. He was still unmarried, and his only close relatives were two brothers in America. They had been sent for, but did not arrive in time for the funeral. He had received the last rites of the Roman Catholic Church, and the body lay in state in Athleague church till Tuesday morning, when Mass was said for his soul, and the funeral started for Roscommon churchyard at two o'clock. It was the largest funeral seen there for many years. Young men marched in procession wearing white sashes and carrying white wands, and the whole district mourned his passing. Aleen was one of several hundreds who attended the funeral.

Obituaries of those days tended to be long and flowery, but it is extraordinary how both the local people and the profession took his death to heart. Editorials in all the veterinary papers conveyed a sense of personal loss that is most unusual, and there was a warmth and affection that glowed from the pages in their accounts of his kindness, his wit, and his career. There was a photograph of him in the *Veterinary Journal*, and a pen and ink sketch in the *Roscommon Messenger*. These showed a pleasant, thoughtful face with a firm chin and a high domed forehead. In the town square of Roscommon there still stands a plain granite monument raised to his memory. It gives his name and dates and a text, and says it was `erected by a few friends in affectionate remembrance´, but hardly anyone in the town today could say what was so special about him. He had made no Will, so his estate went to the American relatives, but Castlestrange, where he had lived and worked for the past twenty years, was left empty. In 1920 it was burnt down by the Republican forces, and is today in ruins.

Aleen had more cause than most to be grateful to him. He had launched her, taught her, and defended her with all the impetuous generosity of his nature, and he was probably the best friend she ever had in the profession. Whether he meant more to her than young Bertram Widdrington, whom she so nearly married in 1904, it is impossible to say, but the sudden loss of such a colleague must have been a severe jolt. However, she ultimately benefitted, in that she succeeded to his practice, and within two years she had purchased a house in the centre of Athleague, and only a few miles from Castlestrange. This house was known as `Fort Lyster'. Today it is totally demolished, but two heavy stone gateposts remain, with the name carved upon them.

In 1911 she kept there a household of two manservants and two maidservants. Some of the older people in Athleague remember Aleen very clearly. She was `a very big woman', `a tall, fine looking woman', `a robust woman' and `a very refined woman'. Her hair - very thick and plentiful to judge by photographs - was `not red, but auburn'.

Mr James Cox, an elderly gentleman still living in Athleague in 1981, was familiar with her daily routine. At work she always wore a long gaberdine skirt and jacket, and a man's wide brimmed hat. She never took breakfast, but during the day she ate oat cakes, and a bunch of fresh watercress, delivered every morning from a spring in the village. She kept many animals of her own - goats, some Jersey cows, some black Kerry cows, and lots of cats and cocker spaniels. Every month or so she would supply goats' milk to the children's hospital in Dublin, nearly a hundred miles away. She generally did her visits on horseback, riding side-saddle, often on a white Arab stallion. If she needed to carry equipment she used a back-to-back gig. If medicines were needed the farmers would usually call at her house for them. In those days the size of a practice was assessed by the number of horses needed to run it. Hers was a `four horse practice' of about seven or eight miles radius. Very few farmers had private telephones, so they used to send for her by telegram. Mr James Waldron, whose father kept the Post Office at Athleague, used as a boy to deliver telegrams to her, often three or four a day. At seven o'clock in the evening, when her day's work was over, she would change and put on `a beautiful ball gown' and sit down to dinner, waited on by her servants.

For wealthy people she would charge one or two pounds for a visit, but she never charged the poorer people anything, and often gave them money instead, when she treated their animals. In the Ireland of those days the distinction between rich and poor was gross and obvious, so this system did not pose the problem that it would in modern cities.

At the appropriate season she would castrate many colts, sometimes dozens at a time being assembled for her. This almost certainly means that she must have `castrated standing´, that is, without casting and giving an anaesthetic. This was the subject of much controversy from the late nineteenth century right up to the nineteen thirties. Experienced and highly skilled veterinary surgeons could perform this operation in a few minutes, with but one skilled assistant, and they claimed that it caused the colt less upset than the terror of being cast and chloroformed. For operators of less experience, or who were not regularly castrating colts, it was a daunting prospect, and if anything went wrong could be highly dangerous to both patient and surgeon. There was always the problem of how many accidents could be suffered while one was acquiring the necessary skill, but Aleen was an excellent surgeon and she had that uncanny knack with horses that engenders trust. Today, with far fewer horses and much better anaesthetics than chloroform, the practice was probably extinct even before it became illegal.

It was this particular operation above all others being done by a woman which scandalized the local priest, and he would have dearly loved to have put a stop to it. Indeed, he urged his flock never to employ Miss Cust, but they continued to do so. One day the priest's own cow became ill, and the villagers were delighted to see Aleen riding through the village in broad daylight on her white horse, to stop and tie up at the priest's house. Animal welfare, especially in Ireland, can sometimes take precedence over the most deeply held prejudices.

There was one operation, rather new to the profession in Britain, which Aleen did not herself attempt as yet, but her friend Professor Hobday had made it his speciality. The nerves to the larynx of the horse have a very complex arrangement and one of them is occasionally affected by a form of paralysis. This makes the vocal cords of one or both sides fall slack and partially obstruct the breathing. A horse so affected makes a characteristic sound at every breath, especially at exercise, and is known as a `roarer´. With good anaesthesia and a dexterious surgeon it is possible to strip out the lining of the space between the vocal cord and the side of the larynx, which causes the cord to adhere in the `open´ position, so that the breathing is no longer obstructed and the condition is permanently cured. Hobday did not

48

invent the operation, but he became very skilled at doing it and went all over the country demonstrating the method. His services were in great demand because he could turn an otherwise worthless horse into a useful hunter, provided the original diagnosis was correct. In October 1910 Hobday was in Ireland and attended a meeting of the Central Veterinary Association of Ireland at Ballinasloe. The Society scrapped its prepared programme to take full advantage of Hobday's presence, and he gave a demonstration of the 'roaring' operation. It was the time of the Ballinasloe Annual Fair - a very great occasion - and Hobday was royally entertained. Aleen was at this meeting and another lady, Miss English, was also present. This lady was a surgeon in human medicine, and the resident medical officer of the local asylum. At the end of of the meeting Mr Winter said they had surgeons there that evening who were not members, two ladies! (cries of `hear hear!´). They were delighted to see them there, and he was sure he spoke the feelings of all when he said it gave the members much pleasure to see these two ladies at the meeting of their Association (loud applause). Mr Winter then gave them the toast of `The Ladies´ which was honoured with great cordiality. Mr Howard, on behalf of the ladies, returned thanks to Mr Winter and the members generally. They had not seen their way to open the door and admit ladies to their ranks. He was waiting to see if the Suffragettes would take up this matter (laughter and applause) and was looking forward to see their esteemed `civic fathers´, the Royal College of Veterinary Surgeons, open its arms (loud applause and laughter) and welcome the ladies (applause).

Thus encouraged, Aleen had Professor Hobday over again in May 1911 specially to perform the roaring operation on a valuable horse belonging to one of her clients. This was in itself an acknowledgment of Aleen's professional status, as etiquette strictly forbids a qualified veterinary surgeon to consult or collaborate with an unqualified person.

In August of that year Aleen's friend Professor Owen Williams, son of her old principal, and now himself principal of the Liverpool School, attended a meeting of the other Veterinary Association of Ireland in Dublin, but Miss Cust was not present and apparently did not meet him. Sixteen days later Owen Williams was dead, at the early age of fifty-one. His health had been weakened by malaria and typhoid, contracted during his army service abroad, but his lively and cheerful disposition made his sudden death an unexpected blow. It was as well for Aleen that she had made so many new friends in the past few years that the deaths of Willie Byrne and Owen Williams could no longer seriously hinder her career, however keenly she may have felt the personal loss.

In October 1913 Miss Cust again read a paper to the Central Veterinary Association of Ireland. This time it was essentially clinical and was entitled 'Several Odd Cases'. It was a good workman-like paper and gave rise to an animated discussion. Reading it today it is evident that there was nothing brilliant or particularly original about it, but in both its content and presentation it was well ahead of many of the more pompous perorations by `eminent practitioners´ of her day. The form she chose - a string of short clinical anecdotes with no thematic connection - was a common one in those days, and was always enjoyed by other practitioners, because there was something for everybody and they could all air their views to their mutual benefit about the problems raised. This time the meeting was fully reported without comment in the *Veterinary Record*. Aleen had indeed arrived in the profession, albeit by the back door.

By this time Aleen was not alone in her aspirations. In July 1913 the RCVS Council had to consider a letter from Thomas H. Greig, of Edinburgh, asking how women could get training as veterinary surgeons. The secretary had already told him that the Council had no legal power to admit women, but while expressing polite thanks for this information Mr Greig persisted:-

> "I will be much obliged now by your being good enough to let me know to whom I shall apply in order to get ladies legally admitted to a course of study and to the examinations necessary to secure a diploma which will enable them to practise the profession of veterinary physicians and surgeons with similar and equally valuable privileges to those granted to successful male students of those subjects. I am not particular at present whether this course and the examinations can be taken in any of the existing colleges, or whether a separate college must be provided for them. That can be arranged afterwards, though I should prefer the use of the existing colleges for the ladies' classes.
>
> Believe me, yours faithfully, etc. etc."

The President invited comments, and Sir Stewart Stockman proposed that it be referred to the Parliamentary Committee for report. He continued:-

"I understand there is a desire amongst some members to have a discussion on it, but, as I pointed out in committee, it is a sleeping dog which was put to rest some years ago by a decision of the Scottish Courts, and when it was put to rest it was done with the acclamation of the members of the profession."

This tactic served to delay matters until January 1914, when the Parliamentary and General Purposes Committee reported by merely repeating the previous opinion that in the Charter of 1844 and the Act of 1881 `students´ at the colleges referred to were male students, and only such persons were the persons to be included. A similar enquiry had also been received from the Veterinary School of Liverpool University.

Mr Thatcher, the College Solicitor, rose to the occasion with a long speech reiterating all that he had said in 1897 about `usage´ making it impossible for the RCVS to admit women to their examinations without a special dispensation from Parliament. One of his trump cards was that the legal profession, his own, also excluded women and had just won a lawsuit about it. A certain Miss Gwyneth Marjorie Bebb had given notice to the Law Society that she wished to take their preliminary examination in February 1913, and had enclosed the requisite fee. The Society had returned the fee and informed her that if she presented herself for examination she would not be admitted, giving the reason that she was a woman, and therefore could not be admitted as a solicitor of the Supreme Court. She had therefore brought an action against the Law Society asking for a *mandamus* directing the defendant Society to admit her to the examination. This had been a test case, and three other young women, equally well qualified, were awaiting the outcome. The action had been dismissed, but Miss Bebb had appealed. In the Court of Appeal the action had been dismissed with costs. The arguments were roughly the same as those used against Miss Cust, but in Miss Bebb's case they had at least been debated in open court instead of the issue being evaded. The legal profession is very much older than the veterinary profession, so they could claim `usage´ going back to the time of Henry IVth, since when no attorney had ever been a woman. In a newspaper report of 1912 Mr E. A. Bell, a solicitor in favour of admitting women in his profession, had said it was necessary

"to register articles entered into with a solicitor by taking them to the Law Society. The Society requires the person to swear that he is of the male sex."

51

Now this was something the RCVS had not thought necessary, probably because they considered themselves sufficiently expert in such matters to judge for themselves. Miss Bebb's case was almost exactly the same as that of Miss Cust, and her losing it set the minds of the RCVS Council at rest at long last. She could no longer claim that if she wished she had a legal right to admission.

But Miss Bebb had several eager colleagues, and all these ladies were expert in legal matters. They immediately set about drafting a Bill to be presented to Parliament at the earliest opportunity `for removing the existing disability' and by February 1914 it was ready for introduction. Had they succeeded it would have been most mortifying for the RCVS, as their own modest Bill, now desperately necessary for their very survival, had already been thrown out after a first reading on three successive occasions. They persevered with it, but this was 1914, and soon all plans were endangered by the cataclysm which so few people in the profession seem to have foreseen. The British veterinary profession was wholly preoccupied by the 10th International Veterinary Congress, which opened in London on 3rd August. When war broke out on the 4th August the few delegates still present dispersed at once.

Unlike those on the Continent the British Government never took such Congresses seriously enough to consider allocating funds for them, and all the expense was borne by the profession. They had been collecting money among themselves for three or four years, and with halls booked in advance and papers printed etc. the expense was almost as great following cancellation as if the Congress had taken place. The loss was even greater from a cultural point of view as these international gatherings were the very life blood of science at a time when regular contacts with colleagues abroad were much fewer and more difficult than today.

However, like everyone else, the veterinary surgeons shrugged off their disappointment and took on the work of `winning the war'.

CHAPTER V

Wartime

"A horse! a horse! my kingdom for a horse!"

Shakespeare - `Richard III'

For those born after the nineteen twenties it may be difficult to appreciate how completely dependent on horses was the preceding civilization. Both public and private transport was almost entirely horse-drawn, and even the railways depended on horse transport to link the railway stations with factories and houses. Buses and trams, fire-engines, the doctor and the humble costermonger all relied on horses or donkeys. In 1897 a strike of farriers threatened to paralyse all London transport, and the situation was only saved by the availability of hundreds of non-union farriers who flooded into the capital from the rural areas.

By 1914 the changes due to mechanization were well under way, and had even introduced a new factor into methods of war, although their full impact was not yet apparent. The guns and supplies could not move except with horses and mules, and the war could not have been waged without them. The War Office calculated that in the event of war they would need, suddenly and immediately, 160,000 horses to augment their peace-time strength of 23,000. Some kind of census of the horse population of the British Isles was needed. At first it was suggested that the police carried this out, but the average policeman's knowledge of horse flesh was considered inadequate for this purpose.

In 1912 Maj. Gen. Sir William Birkbeck, popularly known as "Brickbat", became Director of Remounts at Army headquarters. He gained a reputation for cheerful, ruthless efficiency in cutting red tape and giving capable men their head. He it was who secretly commissioned a certain Col. MacMunn, and a small team of like-minded colleagues to locate the necessary horses and devise means of acquiring them at once when, but not before, the necessity arose. Some enabling legislation was quietly slipped through Parliament, and the team made their own census and laid plans for the requisition of horses as

53

required. Some details of how they achieved this were revealed nearly forty years later in the *Journal of the Royal Artillery* of 1950 by Lt. Gen. Sir George MacMunn, as he had become by then. Their schemes worked because they understood horses and horse owners, and treated them fairly but firmly. Not more than half an individual owner's stud was requisitioned without consent, and reasonable prices were paid on the spot. The omnibus companies were just beginning to change over to motorbuses, and full advantage of this was taken to horse the artillery. When the supply of horses from the British Isles was exhausted they already knew the most fruitful sources abroad, and before the war was over the Army had purchased horses from Europe, America and Australia. The world-wide extent of the British Empire facilitated this and gave the Allies a marked advantage over the enemy.

Having acquired all these animals it was up to the small veterinary profession to maintain them in a state fit for the arduous conditions of the fighting line. In the Boer war, twelve to fifteen years earlier, our forces had been gravely hampered by poor organisation of the Remount and Veterinary services. The War Office had by now learned that particular lesson. The Remount Service was in the capable hands of "Brickbat" and a new body, the Army Veterinary Corps had been formed. Previously, veterinary surgeons had been attached as individuals to various cavalry regiments. Now they were a 'Corps', consisting of 767 officers and 16,400 men, under Maj. Gen. Sir John Moore, as Director of Veterinary Services with the British Expeditionary Force in France. Birkbeck's deputy in France was Brig. Gen. F. S. Garratt, Director of Remounts. It was essential that the sick and injured horses were at all times separate from the fit and healthy, yet there was such a constant interchange between categories that the two departments necessarily worked in close collaboration all the time.

General Moore was in charge of the field hospitals, six to begin with, each accommodating 250 horses. By 1917 this had risen to eighteen hospitals and four convalescent depots, accommodating in all nearly 40,000 animals. Apart from the veterinary surgeons employed in the hospitals the rest of the Corps were organised in 'mobile sections'. These were small teams of about ten veterinary surgeons, with other ranks assisting. They were supplied with motor horse ambulances by the RSPCA, who assiduously collected money for these in England. Immediately after every action a mobile section would swoop into the battlefield, shoot any horses too badly hurt for treatment, and remove those less seriously injured for evacuation to the hospitals. This kept the front lines clear of unuseable horses, while those suitable for treatment went back to base by rail, road or barge as was most convenient. There was a constant flow of supplies of food and ammunition up to the front, and the empty waggons were used to evacuate the horses. Human casualties in the Veterinary Corps were much lighter than in the units in the front line, but the work was arduous, highly skilled, and often for very long hours.

Thousands of animals were constantly arriving at the Channel Ports, where they would be examined, rested, and any sick ones weeded out before they were sent to the front. Simultaneously sick and wounded animals were constantly being evacuated to the base hospitals, where they were sorted into infectious and non-infectious cases and treated appropriately. As soon as they were regarded as `cured' they went to convalescent depots, as it was no good sending them up to the front until they had been got into training again with good food and graded exercise. Conditions at the front were often so bad that horses were driven to exhaustion and had to be evacuated to convalescent depots to be rested and given regular food and water until they recovered.

Occasionally there would be a hue and cry because a case of glanders had been detected. This is a chronic disease of horses which is infective for human beings, and in those days the disease in human beings was usually fatal. It was dying out in Britain, but occurred on the Continent, and occasionally in purchases from abroad. All Army horses were regularly tested for this disease, and the occurrence of a `positive' test meant that perhaps a whole shipload might have to be isolated and retested before it was safe to issue them to the front, where they would be in intimate contact with the troops. It is an interesting example of war psychosis that the veterinary staff of both the Allied and German armies suspected that the other side had deliberately spread this disease among their opponents' horses. There is no official mention of such a policy being pursued by either side, but at least one suspicious incident has been reliably reported, and this was probably due to local and unofficial initiative.

Several times the rations had to be cut. Forage is bulky stuff, and either from a genuine shortage or from false economy or mismanagement the amounts would be reduced. This resulted in numerous cases of `debility' within a few weeks or months, as horses could not work unless well fed, and work at the front was always hard.

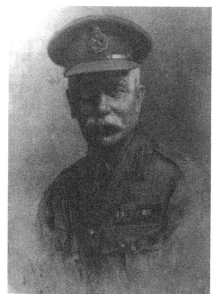

Brigadier General F. S. Garratt

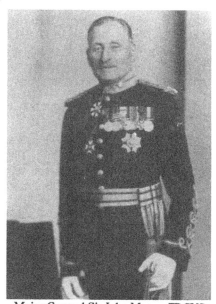

Major General Sir John Moore, FRCVS

Somehow the new Veterinary Corps coped with all this - a nightmare of thousands of horses and mules coming and going at all hours and requiring urgent decisions as to which went where; and a moment's negligence would spell disaster. Horses broke loose and stampeded; horses were mysteriously delayed on the railway and left without food or water; horses were injured by careless shunting, or lost at sea by storms or submarine action; General X's favourite charger, treated for some trivial complaint, had been inadvertently issued to someone else; Sergeant Y, an invaluable groom and dresser, was drunk on night duty; Captain Z had allowed his hospital to get into a filthy and unhygienic condition. All these worries and emergencies, great and small, found their way to General Moore's office, and he and his staff dealt with them. Moore must have been an organising genius and singularly imperturbable. He lasted the whole duration of the war, and afterwards wrote a book about it. His Corps were a motley collection including both newly qualified fledgelings and practitioners who ought to have been considered over-age for the Army. There were a few illustrious names, including Professor Hobday, who had recently been lecturing in surgery to the man who was now his Commanding Officer, and young Lt. Dalling - full of ideas about equine pathology - who rose to be a Major, and in later life became Director of the Ministry of Agriculture's veterinary research. The new Corps won its spurs and proved its worth. The British Army had a lower `wastage´ rate of horses than any of its allies or its enemies. In the early years of the war they had a `cure and re-issue´ rate of 84%, but this fell to 78% as the war progressed and the quality of available horses deteriorated.

In November 1918 His Majesty King George Vth was pleased to grant his new Army Veterinary Corps the prefix `Royal´ and it has been the Royal Army Veterinary Corps ever since.

But where in all this hurlyburly was Aleen Cust? Officially she did not exist for most of the time. Unofficially rumours are multiple and contradictory. Her cousin's son thinks she may have been actually in charge of a Remount Depot in France. She said she worked in one, and also in the veterinary laboratory, but the War Office has no knowledge of this.

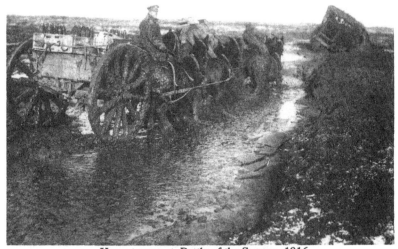

Horse transport, Battle of the Somme, 1916

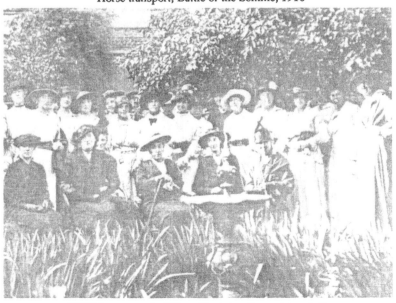

YMCA personnel. ?Aleen Cust standing extreme left

58

Just before the war, in June 1914, Lady Cust had died at the age of seventy-nine. Aleen seems to have had no contact with her mother since she left home to become a veterinary surgeon. Nevertheless Lady Cust did leave her a share of her money, but all her jewellery, lace, and personal effects went to Ursula, Aleen's younger sister. The household property - furniture, silver, carriages, etc. were left to Ursula and her brother Leopold. Neither of these two ever married, and after their mother's death they lived together in a large secluded house in Surrey, with a male nurse for the ailing Leopold and Lady Cust's former maid as a companion for Ursula. Lady Corbet, a wealthy aunt with whom the family often stayed after Sir Leopold's death, also died on the day before war broke out, so such family ties as Aleen had were fast dissolving.

For a year she remained in her practice in Athleague. Local practitioners were much involved in the selection and evaluation of horses for requisitioning, and Aleen's knowledge of local conditions and personalities would have been much in demand. The Army found more and better horses in Ireland than anywhere else in the British Isles, and it was said that the very best of them came from the Roscommon area, where Aleen reigned. However, by the spring of 1915 the supply of Irish horses was all but exhausted, and the Army was turning to America and Canada. Aleen was involved in a minor lawsuit against a young man who had borrowed her car without permission and crashed it while joy-riding. She won her case, but it was obvious from the judge's comments that his sympathies were with the unfortunate young man, and he thought Aleen's claim for damages excessive. With her best patients requisitioned, and many of her male friends and colleagues enlisted, she felt isolated and disenchanted and longed to be where the action was.

The Army would not have dreamed of using her officially, but with her usual persistence and ingenuity she got to France, with her own car, under the auspices of the Young Men's Christian Association. This organisation did invaluable work during the war. They set out to cater for the spiritual needs of the soldiers, but this was so broadly interpreted that their dedicated organisers found themselves providing everything from writing paper to table tennis, along with endless supplies of hot tea and cocoa and sandwiches. To Christians and atheists alike their premises became a refuge from the cold, the noise, and all the impersonal idiocy of war. They managed to install portable huts in the most unlikely places, and wherever the soldiers were, the YMCA appeared, bringing moral support and a whiff of civilised values.

In the north-east corner of France, inland from Boulogne and Dieppe, were located most of the veterinary hospitals, convalescent homes and

Remount Depots. Both Maj. Gen. Sir John Moore and Brig. Gen. Garratt had their headquarters at Abbeville, from where they were constantly on the move inspecting and advising in their scattered premises. Near Abbeville was a large YMCA hut to cater for the hard-working personnel of these places, where hundreds of horses amd mules were coming and going day and night. This hut was known as the Remount Hut, and it was here that Aleen got herself stationed. She was now a motherly figure of forty-seven, and she probably knew as much about horses as anyone in France. She was also extremely charming, and very fluent in English, French, and German. No doubt she did her full stint of handing out cocoa and sandwiches, but it is inconceivable that she did not also inveigle the harassed young men into talking shop. They would have found her a good listener and a mine of information, and it seems probable that she wheedled her way into the stables and hospital wards for many of her off-duty hours. No hint of this activity was allowed to ruffle the official consciousness, and to senior veterinary surgeons she would have been at best a tiresome old woman and at worse a scandalous anomaly.

Yet the hospitals were chronically short of staff, and the veterinary surgeons they had were grossly overworked. With her long-practised mixture of charm and discretion Aleen may well have been enjoying herself in the exercise of her professional skill behind the official back. There is no positive confirmation of this suspicion, but there is one interesting reference to her in Brigadier General Garratt's war diary. His official war diary is a model of brevity and lucidity. He seldom used any overtly forceful language, although he was obviously a man of strong opinions. He was always meticulous in noting the full name, with initials, rank, or in the case of civilians the precise status and designation of any visitor to his office, and there were many of these. His entry for the 16th November 1916 is as follows:

> "*11a.m. Application made in person* by Miss Cust, Y.M.C.A., for use of draught animals for Y.M.C.A. purposes.
>
> Informed her that any such application must be sent by the head of the Y.M.C.A. to I.G.C. or 2.M.G. G.H.2. It is possible to loan animals fit for use at the base only, if they were fed and stabled, and looked after by Y.M.C.A. personnel, provided the necessary authority was obtained."

The underlining of the first phrase, and the uncharacteristically erratic punctuation, suggest that the General was somewhat disturbed by this encounter. That she is merely `Miss Cust, YMCA´ suggests he knew the lady by reputation only too well, although not used to meeting her `in person´. With the constantly shifting population of horses there were inevitably times when one class of animal predominated. Previous entries in his diary suggest that at that time there was a surplus of semi-recovered horses that were capable of light work and in need of exercise. Aleen, with her ear to the ground, or rather to the floor-boards of the Remount hut, would have known this, and had the temerity to make what seemed to her a sensible suggestion, but evidently the General would have none of it. This is probably typical of most Army Generals of that time, but I suspect she got on better with the lower ranks, both officers and men.

The next official mention of Aleen that has been traced is in the war diary of Major General Sir John Moore, the Director of Veterinary Services in France. He was concerned about Captain E. A. Watson, of the Canadian Army Veterinary Corps, who had been seconded to his department in January 1917 as an expert bacteriologist, to do research work, and also to prepare vaccines as necessary. He had a small laboratory at Rouen, provided by the RSPCA, but he needed larger premises and some skilled assistance. On the 19th September 1917, Moore suggested that there should be a new laboratory, staffed by a bacteriologist with the rank of Major, an assistant with the rank of Captain, a laboratory superintendent with the rank of Sergeant, and four assistants (women).

All this seems to have been too much for the War Office, for on the 16th November 1917, he makes a more modest suggestion:

"I am of the opinion that much of the routine work could be carried out as well, if not better, by women than by men. I have accordingly written to Miss Aileen (sic) Cust, who has completed the curriculum in a veterinary college, suggesting that she should apply to be enrolled, and given a suitable grading in the W.A.A.C., when it would probably be arranged that she should be detailed for work in the laboratory. I think there would be no difficulty in obtaining other women who were also suited for the work. Miss Cust would not appear to consider the suggestion to be free from objection, but I am again writing to her."

Sir John had been stationed in Ireland for some years before the war, and frequently attended meetings of the Irish Central Veterinary Society, so he must have known Aleen at least by repute, and was probably a personal acquaintance. It would be interesting to know just how Aleen phrased her misgivings about this offer. There is no evidence that she had any bent for bacteriology, or more than a superficial interest in the subject. Many veterinary surgeons of that era hardly ever used a microscope except for the occasional examination of skin scrapings for mange parasites, and the chances are that she had not done any serious bacteriological work since leaving college in 1900. The assumption that someone whose major pre-occupation for seventeen years had been clinical work with horses and cattle would automatically, because of her sex, be suited to `routine bacteriology´ is a strange one, but this idea occurred repeatedly among male veterinary surgeons until well into the nineteen forties. Of course many veterinary surgeons, both male and female, do make excellent bacteriologists, but by no means all have either the desire or the gift for it. However, Aleen was neat fingered and quick witted, and could probably adapt to new work better than most. It would seem that patriotism, or the possible chance of advancemnent, triumphed, and in January 1918 Aleen duly enlisted in the Queen Mary's Army Auxiliary Corps.

The War Office gives her dates as the 14th January to the 10th November 1918, and says she served in France from the 10th February to the 9th October. These dates suggest that she returned to England to enlist, and then went out again to France. On the 13th February, three days after she was officially in France, the Commanding Officer of the QMAAC in Rouen notes that `Miss A. Cust, Unit Administrator from Abbeville´ arrived.

Rank in the QMAAC was complicated by a phobia of the War Office lest anybody, least of all the women themselves, should consider them part of the Army, or in any way equivalent to proper male soldiers. During the second World War they gradually got over this, and a less mystifying nomenclature was used, but in 1918 no woman could be called by any designation of rank which was also used by men. Dame Helen Gwynne-Vaughan, in her fascinating history of the Corps, gives a table in one of the appendices which explains the equivalents. Thus the lowest rank, corresponding to a Private in the Army, was called a `Worker´. `Sergeant´ became a `Forewoman´, `2nd Lieutenant´ equals `Assistant Administrator´ and `Captain´ a `Unit Administrator´, which is what Miss Cust had now become. Whether she went to Abbeville by accident or intention (and if so whose?) is not revealed, but she may possibly have had an interview with Major General Moore between the 10th and 13th February, though he does not mention her again in his official diary.

Neither does anyone else mention her in the available documents. Moreover other women stationed at Rouen during the period of Aleen's service have no knowledge of her. A certain Mrs Curtis, who was in her eighty-eighth year in 1984, had a very clear memory of her war service in Rouen. She had been going to the annual reunions of the Corps for many years, but in 1984 there were only seven of them left, so they decided to discontinue the reunions. At this final one she kindly enquired of the others about Aleen, and none of them remembered meeting her. In 1983 a paragraph had been put in the Journal of the Women's Corps (now the A.T.S.) appealing for information about her, but with no result. In view of Aleen's advanced age, compared with her peers in the Corps, and her flamboyant personality, it seems unlikely that she would have escaped notice. It therefore seems probable that she was not employed in the office at Rouen, where most of the other women were, so she may well have been sent to Captain Watson's laboratory.

Whatever her duties were, the appointment seems to have been a disaster. On the 7th July 1918, the Officer in Command of the Rouen station notes in her diary:

> "Interview with D.V.S. reference disposal of Unit Administrator Cust. Instructed to suggest Miss Cust applying for relief from her duties which are not congenial to her."

There must have been very many men and women in all kinds of war service whose duties by that time were not congenial to them, but for whom there was no way out. She was given her campaign medals, so evidently no disgrace was attached to her departure, but the wording is curious. Why should they need to `dispose of´ a Unit Administrator who had apparently committed no misconduct, and was not granted sick leave? The most likely explanation is a clash of personalities. There were no women in the Canadian veterinary profession until 1928, and Captain Watson may have been quite unused to working with women and fiercely resentful of them. He had wanted an assistant, and no doubt assumed it would be a man from the Veterinary Corps. To be fobbed off with an elderly woman who claimed to have trained as a veterinary surgeon while he was still a schoolboy may have been too much for him to stomach. There are occasions when even charm and tact such as Aleen's are of no avail; but since she had been specifically recruited for this post and taken off other war work to fill it, Moore probably felt some responsibility for her and contrived an honourable exit. For another four months she was officially in the Corps, but she left France in October and her engagement finally terminated the day before Armistice Day. Aleen was now fifty, and the conditions in France may well have undermined her previously robust health. The enigmatic termination of her career in the QMAAC must have been a humiliating blow, after which she needed rest and recuperation. She may have found this in the home of her cousin, Mrs Kathleen Skipwith, the daughter of Lady Cust's sister Leila. Some time after the war Aleen became extremely ill and nearly died of pneumonia, and it was Kathleen who nursed her through this at her own home in London. Her stay in the Skipwith household cemented a lasting friendship with Kathleen's son, who rose to become Commander Skipwith in the Navy. Some years later, when Aleen was advised to go to a warmer climate for the winter, she stayed in Spain for several months while Commander Skipwith's ship was at Gibraltar. He says she `liked the Navy´ and used to attend parties on board ship. The old charm never deserted her, and it would seem that the Navy liked her.

CHAPTER VI

`A Matter of Plain Justice´

"...till the multitude make virtue of the faith they had denied"

J. Russell Lowell

Meanwhile, back in England, the Council of the Royal College of Veterinary Surgeons continued with its quarterly meetings, struggling, in spite of the stress of war to maintain their standards - academic, professional, and, not least, standards of propriety. Under the last heading they regarded the question of the admission of women to their ranks. Sir John McFadyean and his son-in-law Sir Stewart Stockman were against it, with an almost religious fervour. Men from the universities, especially that of Liverpool, which was unique in that it actually housed one of the five veterinary colleges, were strongly in favour. Other members of the Council wavered, not so much desiring the change as appreciating that the RCVS was beginning to look old fashioned, almost ridiculous, in its opposition.

Enquiries had been made, and fobbed off with dignity and firmness, as far back as 1913, but the assault was renewed in May 1915, when the Registrar of Liverpool wrote asking whether in the event of women attending the necessary course in veterinary subjects at Liverpool University, the Council of the College would be prepared to admit such candidates to their examinations, and, if successful, to issue to them licences to practise. He was duly informed by the Parliamentary and General Purposes Committee that the Council had no power to admit women. When the Committee reported this to the full Council Mr Share-Jones, who was on the staff of the Liverpool Veterinary College, asked if "the solicitor would give us, very briefly, the grounds upon which that advice is based".

The stalwart Mr Thatcher, while constitutionally incapable of brevity, brought up his heavy artillery and explained at great length how the medical profession had needed a special Act of Parliament to enable *them* to admit women; and how in his own profession Miss Bebb had lost the case that she brought against the Law Society on precisely

65

similar grounds; and that owing to the Veterinary Surgeon's Charter of 1844, to say nothing of the Highland and Agricultural Society of Scotland's agreement of 1856, and the fact that the lady who essayed to be admitted to the RCVS examinations in 1897 had made no attempt to pursue the case when the RCVS had contested it, and that since then none of the veterinary colleges had admitted women to the course, it was proved it was not merely undesirable but impossible.

Nevertheless Mr Share-Jones, with relentless logic, pointed out that all modern universities admitted women to all their courses, and that London University gave a degree in Veterinary Science which any woman was free to take.

McFadyean protested that this was not a degree in Veterinary Science but a simple `B.Sc.´ with (Veterinary Science) in brackets after it. If a woman were to take such a course she could not use it as a licence to practice, and if she did the RCVS would prosecute her.

Share-Jones was unconvinced, and would have continued the argument, but the President of the College, F. W. Garnett, came to McFadyean's rescue with "I cannot allow this discussion to continue". So the RCVS was saved for the Patriarchy, but the victory was precarious.

Share-Jones, who gained his doctorate in Veterinary Science later that summer, had distinctly advanced views on women in the professions, possibly because his wife had, in 1914, become the first woman to have a degree in law, gaining her LLB with First Class Honours at Liverpool University. He had publicised his views in an address to a conference of University women at Sheffield, at which he argued that there was no reason why any branch of veterinary work should be unsuitable for women, as skill rather than strength was required, and he hoped the RCVS would soon admit women.

The Veterinary Record of 31/7/1915 published without comment a quotation from *The Animals' Guardian* which castigated Share-Jones as an impractical academic who had no idea of the rigours of veterinary work. On the other hand *The Times* - that bastion of orthodoxy - had on 22/4/1915 published the following paragraph:-

> `In view of the recognition of women in the medical services, and the rank of Major bestowed on Dr Garrett-Anderson for her work at the military hospital which she and Dr Flora Murray are opening in Endall Street, it is curious to find that the RCVS still refuse to admit women. The matter was recently referred by the College to their solicitor and he decided that as only men students

were admitted at the time the Charter was granted, only men students could be admitted in future. The number of veterinary surgeons is not very large, only about 3,400 being on the Register, and the demand from the Army and the Civil Authorities appears to be greater than the supply.'

In February 1918 yet another request came from Liverpool. In certain cases where a qualification in Agriculture was held, students were sometimes allowed exemption from part or all of the first year of the RCVS Diploma Course. The Examination Committee was asked to consider an application from Miss E. G. Knight, who was about to take the final examination for a Diploma in Agriculture from Reading Agricultural College. The usual stone-walling reply was given about the Council not having the power to admit women, but they had not heard the last of Miss Knight.

In April 1919 an Editorial in the *Veterinary Record*, reporting on the work of the Parliamentary Committee of the RCVS, said that "as was inevitable, the question of admitting women to the profession has been revived and is to be further considered by the Council". Miss Knight had again applied to the Examination Committee, but this time they had replied that "no decision was possible at present". The reason for this slight change of emphasis was revealed in the minutes of the full Council meeting of 11/4/1919. Many time-honoured attitudes and ideas were changing, and the law of the land was beginning to catch up with some of these changes. The Secretary called the attention of Council to Clause I of the Women's Emancipation Bill now before Parliament, which provided for the removal of the Sex Disqualification, and it was resolved that the matter should be referred to the Annual Fee Committee. This committee was struggling to get through Parliament the contentious Veterinary Surgeon's Act (Amendment) Bill which was designed to rescue them from impending bankruptcy by enabling them to charge an annual fee to all veterinary surgeons on the Register. They had been trying to get this legislation passed since 1911, but so far it had never got further than a first reading in Parliament. The Annual Fee Committee decided that no alteration of their proposed Bill was necessary, and referred the matter back to the Council. However, at the next quarterly meeting, on 3/7/1919, the Solicitor pointed out that the `Women's Qualification Bill' as he called it, was coming up for the Report stage in Parliament, and they could really do nothing unless and until it became law. It was agreed that the matter stand over till the next Council meeting.

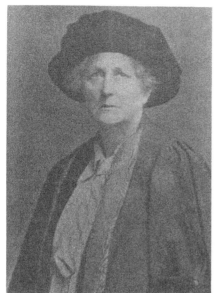

Aleen Cust in Academic Dress, circa 1927

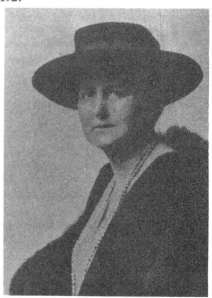

Aleen Cust, studio portrait. Date unknown

68

When this meeting was held on 10/10/1919 the Bill concerning women had still not been passed into law, although the proposed text was available, having been passed by the House of Lords in August. The Secretary drew the attention of the Parliamentary Committee of the Council to the wording, which unequivocally forbade the exclusion of women from any profession merely on grounds of their sex. The full Council therefore sought to discuss it.

Mr J. McKinna was now President of the RCVS, and he opened the discussion by asking Mr Garnett if he had anything to add with reference to this item. Despite his opposition a few years previously Mr Garnett had shifted his ground in the light of changing circumstances. He foresaw the inevitable passing of this law, which would compel the admission of women into all the professional bodies, including the RCVS. He therefore proposed that any woman who presented herself under the existing rules should be examined. He added that "of course the option remains with the Schools as to whether they will teach them or not, but if they do not teach them I think it is quite within the limits of probability that there will be a Women's Veterinary College." Mr Mulvey seconded the resolution. He thought it would be a more graceful act to admit them now rather than wait until they were forced to do so.

Sir John McFadyean rose "to move the previous question" - a formal device to prevent further discussion - although he himself continued to expound his opinion. He said:-

"It is not wise to pass a resolution like this. It is cowardly to do it, because you are only doing it because you think women *will* be admitted. I can mention a much more solid reason for steadying your hands, and that is that such matters as the admission of women to this profession ought not to be settled by the opinions of members of this Council but by the profession - which has never been consulted. I challenge anybody to say that he knows that a majority of the profession are in favour of the admission of women, and they will not thank you for having admitted them at the present time."

He again moved the "previous question". McFadyean's son-in-law Sir Stewart Stockman, seconded the motion, saying:-

> "I think we can quite well wait until this becomes law. When it becomes law we are obliged to accept them, and why draw attention to it now and invite these ladies to come in?"

Mr Mulvey:

> "Because we have already got applications from lady candidates."

Sir Stewart Stockman:

> "Then let them wait until the thing is law.

The President asked for the Solicitor's opinion, and Mr Thatcher said (at great length) that it was absolutely *ultra vires* for them to pass a resolution admitting women to the examinations, which seemed to settle it. But Mr Garnett was not satisfied and asked permission to speak again. He insisted that if it were illegal to admit women, and Council nevertheless passed a resolution to do so, it would be up to those who opposed it to apply for an injunction to restrain Council from admitting women. He added that if this did happen "I will guarantee, no matter how much money they have at their backs, they cannot get a Court of Law to substantiate their position".

Sir Stewart Stockman:

> "Why raise that position at all?"

McFadyean now waded in afresh:

> "With respect to veterinary matters in many affairs I attach great importance to the opinion of Mr Garnett, but when the question is one of law I prefer the opinion of our Solicitor, and I move the previous question."

The President said lamely:

> "I think the thing falls to the ground now"

and Mr Garnett withdrew his resolution.

The Bill did eventually become law on the 23rd December 1919, and went under the somewhat strange title of `The Sex Disqualification

(Removal) Act´. It provided that a person shall not be disqualified by sex or marriage from `assuming or carrying on any civil profession or vocation, or for admission to any incorporated Society (whether incorporated by Royal Charter or otherwise)´.

At the next quarterly meeting of the RCVS Council on 9th January 1920 the Secretary brought it to their notice, and the Solicitor - in one of his shortest speeches ever recorded - said "That is so. Women are now entitled to enter the veterinary profession". Mr Mulvey said they had already had an application, and it had been passed. This presumably referred to Miss Edith Knight, who in October 1920 was admitted to the Liverpool Veterinary College as a second year student, having been granted exemption of most of the first year subjects because of her Agricultural Diploma.

A cautious editorial in the *Veterinary Record* of 24/1/1920 noted the passage of the Act but added "it need not concern us greatly, for it is not likely that women will offer themselves in sufficient numbers to be of serious moment". However, Mr W. T. D. Broad, President of the Royal Counties Division of the National Veterinary Medical Association (predecessor of the British Veterinary Association) reviewing the manpower situation in the profession said gloomily "Africa is about to train her own, and our members will probably be increased by the entrance of the fair sex soon - without the Royal College having any say in the matter". Within a year Dublin Veterinary College also admitted women students, but it was years before the Scottish and London Colleges did so. The first examination results which included women candidates recorded that Miss Knight had passed her second year or `Class B´ examination with Second Class Honours, which was an excellent beginning.

Edith Gertrude Knight had come by a spartan route into the Veterinary Course. Nearly thirty years younger than Miss Cust, she had started her career as a private pupil to a woman farmer, because she wanted an open air life with animals. During the war her employer had to be absent for a time, and she ran the whole hundred acre farm with very little help. It involved long hours and much heavy work. Her father thought her health was deteriorating and persuaded her to leave and obtain proper training at Reading Agricultural College. She gained the Diploma in Agriculture in 1918, and stayed on at Reading for a year as a research assistant. Thanks to her combination of practical experience and scientific aptitude she did particularly useful work in some classical experiments on the production of bacteriologically `clean´ milk. Like Miss Cust she loved horses, being an inveterate rider to hounds, and she

71

used to help exercise the horses belonging to G. P. Male, a highly respected veterinary surgeon in practice at Reading. He was a part-time lecturer to the students at Reading Agricultural College, where Miss Knight first came to his notice, and it was he who suggested she would make a good veterinary surgeon. She was more than willing, but said she understood they would not have women. "Well" he said "that may be changing". From then on she set her sights on a veterinary career.

As already mentioned she began making applications to the RCVS in 1918, and after the Bill was passed there was no stopping her. In fact she might easily have completed the course and herself been the first woman on the Register, which would have been a wry humiliation for Aleen Cust, who had been soldiering on since 1900 in the teeth of official opposition of the RCVS, the Ministry of Agriculture, and the Army.

Aleen was now back in Ireland, attempting to pick up the war torn threads of her old practice in Athleague. Willie Byrne was dead, General Moore was in India, and many of her Irish friends and colleagues were dead or scattered. Moreover the Ireland she knew was changing rapidly. During the years of her absence the Easter Rising had occurred and been defeated. This was followed by the Anglo-Irish war. In December 1921 an uneasy peace was signed and the Irish Free State established, omitting six counties to the North. De Valera continued to lead armed resistance until 1923 and refused to co-operate with the new Parliament, so that the country was in a state of civil war that only gradually subsided.

Before the war Aleen's nationality does not seem to have hindered her acceptance by the Irish farming community, and rich and poor alike loved and respected her. Now that she had returned from war service the English aristocrat suddenly found herself regarded as an enemy. Her house was besieged by the Irish Liberation Army, and on at least one occasion she is said to have held them off with a shotgun. For the rest of her life, even when safe in the peace of Hampshire, she always insisted on the curtains being tightly drawn after dark, as a remembered precaution against snipers. The Irish Liberation Army did not harm her person, but they confiscated her car. She told a friend that she did not mind that so much but she was truly grieved when they took her horse whip. Amateur psychologists' hearts may leap up at this remark, but the whip could well have been a keepsake from her father, or from Willie Byrne, or from one of the Widdringtons.

But she still had at least one firm friend in the veterinary profession, and this was Major Frederick Hobday, now running a fashionable small animal practice in the West End of London. He had been a Council member before the war, and was at one time on the staff of the Royal

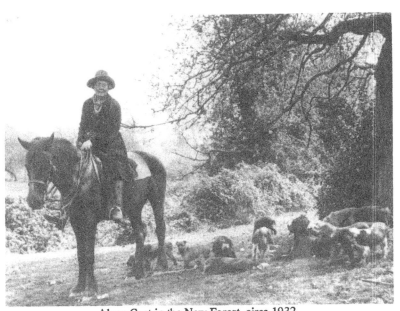

Aleen Cust in the New Forest, circa 1932

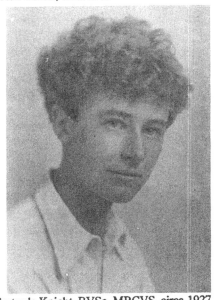

Miss Edith Gertrude Knight, BVSc, MRCVS, circa 1927

73

Veterinary College of London, and he was always in the thick of veterinary politics.

It may well have been he who alerted Aleen to the changed circumstances following the 1919 Act. Hobday would have noted the progress of Miss Knight, and the various other women students at Dublin and Liverpool, as he was an examiner for the RCVS. Knight was due to take her finals in 1923, but in October 1922 Aleen applied to the RCVS Examination Committee for permission to present herself in December 1922 for the final examination, Class D under the four year course. Her application was supported by various testimonials, and by the certified account of her four years training in Edinburgh from 1896 to 1900. Students with war service were being granted various concessions to facilitate completion of interrupted careers, and it was in this category that she applied for the concession. The Examination Committee decided that she need sit only the Oral Examination of the final year.

An Editorial in the *Veterinary Record* of 28th October 1922 unequivocally approved this decision "as a matter of plain justice" and congratulated the Council, extending to Miss Cust "our best wishes for her final success". The London examination results were published in the *Veterinary Record* of 23rd December 1922, and there in the final year, with seven men's names, was the name of Aleen Cust. Henry Sumner was now President of the RCVS, and it was from his hands, on the 21st December 1922, that Aleen received her long coveted Diploma. Mr Sumner had supported the entry of women for some years, and he welcomed her as the first woman to become a veterinary surgeon, saying it marked an epoch in the history of the RCVS.

Then, after twenty-three years of official obloquy, came the tributes and acknowledgments. A long paragraph in the *Veterinary Record* giving details of her career, and stating that she had `served for four years with H. M. Forces during the recent war`; a gracious reference to her in the New Year message from the President of the RCVS to the profession; and a laudatory half-column in *The Field*. This last added a note of caution, however, regarding Miss Cust a wholly exceptional, saying:

> "One swallow does not make a summer, nor does one lady with exceptional physical endowments prove that the veterinary profession is one suitable for women."

The *Veterinary Record* reprinted *The Field*'s article in its issue of 13th January 1923, commenting that it was "something of a relief" after "so much ill-informed eulogistic reference in the lay press since the welcome advent of the first woman veterinary surgeon." Strange to say these `eulogistic articles´ have proved impossible to trace, although Miss Cust's success was reported, briefly, in most of the national daily papers. All these included in their reports the fact that she was the daughter of Sir Leopold Cust and the sister of Sir Charles Cust, equerry to the King. That Leopold had been dead for forty years and Charlie Cust was not on speaking terms with Aleen made no difference to their importance in defining her status.

That week also saw the launching of the first woman barrister, the first woman solicitor, and the first woman architect;   so the Sex Disqualification (Removal) Act was indeed bearing fruit.

Having passed the examination in December 1922 Miss Cust was too late to be included in the 1923 Register, so her name first appeared in the Register of 1924. Her address was given as `c/o Messrs Collyer Bristow and Company, 4 Bedford Row, WC1´. The date of qualification was December 1922, but the place of training was given as `New Edinburgh´. This was true, as all her training had been at this College, although the `New Edinburgh College´ had been moved to Liverpool in 1904, and she actually took the examination at the Royal Veterinary College, London.

The address is that of her solicitors, and she was at that time living in London in some Mews at the back of Eaton Square. Her friends put on a reception for her to celebrate her success, but her sister and brothers refused to attend it. However, the profession was now enthusiastic in its welcome.   The Mid-West and South Wales Veterinary Association, meeting at Bath on 11th January 1923, learned that their secretary, J. J. Aveston, had sent a wire to Miss Cust congratulating her on her admission and inviting her to be present at that meeting. She had replied, thanking him, and saying that but for a previous engagement she would have had much pleasure in accepting, and that she hoped to attend on some future occasion. The Central Veterinary Society, at their meeting in London on the 1st February, nominated her for membership, and she was duly elected at their next meeting on the 1st March. Later in that month at a meeting of the Yorkshire Division of the NVMA Lt. Col. H. G. Bowes, in his presidential address, welcomed the admission of women and said it was `a pleasing coincidence that the first lady to gain the Diploma was the same lady who applied for and was refused permission to sit for the examinations some twenty-odd years ago´.

At the April meeting of the Central Veterinary Society Aleen was present, and was officially welcomed by the President as their first lady member.   She replied, thanking them, and said she had only just

75

succeeded in living long enough to become a member of the profession, and she hoped to be present often at the meetings. The NVMA Annual Congress in September was at York that year, but Miss Cust was not present, and she also sent apologies for her absence at the October meeting of the Central division. At this meeting it was suggested that an informal smoking concert should be held, but Professor Wooldridge demurred, reminding them that they now had a lady member. A few weeks later the *Veterinary Record* contained the following letter from Miss Cust:

`Sir,

Referring to p. 784 of the *Veterinary Record*, which has only just reached me, I want to express my appreciation and gratitude for the thoughtfulness displayed towards me at the meeting of the Central Division of the NVMA. But I would like, at the same time, to make it known that I do not wish to stand in the way of any arrangements, smoking or social, that might be wished for; in fact I sometimes smoke myself - when I can get the right brand of cigarette. In any case I do not suppose that it will be feasible for me to attend the meetings very regularly, as I am not living in London.

Yours faithfully,
Aleen Cust.´

No address was given, but it is probable she had gone back to Ireland for a time to sort out her affairs there.

In December 1923 Miss Knight passed her final examination at Liverpool and became the second British woman to qualify as a veterinary surgeon. She stayed on at Liverpool University, continuing her studies, until in December 1926 she became the first woman to hold the degree of Bachelor of Veterinary Science. This degree was only open to students who were already MRCVS, and it was regarded as a suitable qualification for a research post. Yet for the next six months she was unable to get work of any kind - a situation that was to confront many women veterinary surgeons in the years to come. No matter how competent and well qualified women were, the vast majority of male veterinary surgeons refused to employ them.

However, Miss Knight was luckier than some, and eventually obtained an assistantship on the South Coast. She was not very happy there, but having got her foot in the door she was able to obtain temporary work as *locum tenens,* which increased her experience and gained her good references. At last she became assistant to Capt. J. R. Barker, of Hereford, with whom she had `seen practice' as a student. He was a very fine practitioner who became famous for his work on certain diseases of cattle. She was very happy there and was able to use her talents to the full. The farmers liked her, and accepted her with an alacrity that surprised her male colleagues. Then, in January 1929 Miss Knight married E. L. Taylor, who had been her fellow student at Liverpool. Like her he was also a B.VSc, and he had decided to specialise in parasitology, a hitherto neglected field of veterinary science. He had studied abroad in France and America, and in 1927 obtained a post at the Ministry of Agriculture Veterinary Research Laboratory, near Weybridge, Surrey. So after her marriage Miss Knight - who still used her maiden name for professional purposes - had to leave her post in Herefordshire and work in Surrey. Like so many others of the first few women veterinary surgeons she decided to set up on her own account.

Within a year her first child was born, and the wits of the profession hailed him as `the first thoroughbred'. He did in fact train as a veterinary surgeon when he was older, but eventually he abandoned the profession of his parents to specialise in physiology, and work in human medicine. Meanwhile Miss Knight's practice flourished, but with the interruptions of childbirth she needed assistance, and had the satisfaction of engaging other women veterinary surgeons as *locums.* A second son was born in 1933 and a third in 1935, by which time she had taken Miss Marjorie Jordan, one of the first women to qualify from London, into partnership. She kept a toe-hold in the practice for a few years more, but the responsibility of a growing family began to take up more and more of her time, and she gradually relinquished the practice to Miss Jordan.

In the autumn of 1927 Major Frederick Hobday became Principal of the Royal Veterinary College, London, in succession to Sir John McFadyean, who retired. Hobday was a man of great enthusiasms, and being an old friend of Aleen Cust's he immediately admitted women students, which Sir John had steadfastly refused to do. He also made public speeches, which were widely reported in the press, maintaining that women were eminently suited to veterinary work, more so than men. This was too much for Sir John, and at the Council meeting of the RCVS in April 1929 he proposed the following resolution:-

"The Council of the RCVS, having had their attention called to recent propaganda intended to induce women to become veterinary surgeons, regret to find that the prospects of success for women in the veterinary profession have been greatly exaggerated.

There is no evidence that the men now on the Register of the RCVS are inadequate in number for the treatment of animals in this country. In this connection no true analogy can be drawn between medical and veterinary practice, as the conditions that naturally incline human patients to prefer a woman doctor do not arise in the case of diseased animals.

The Council of the RCVS are bound to disregard the sex of students who present themselves for the diploma of membership, but they feel they would be doing less than their duty if they did not make public their opinion that, in competition with men, women in the veterinary profession will always be under most serious disadvantages and that, in consequence, there can be no justification for the exaggerated prospects of professional success that have been advanced in the public press as an inducement to women to enter the veterinary profession."

This provoked a heated debate. Professor Whitehouse, Principal of the Glasgow Veterinary College, pointed out that some women could in fact do all the usual work of veterinary surgeons perfectly competently, although the prejudices of employers might create difficulties for them at present. Sir John Moore begged them not to pass this resolution as it would be used as propaganda by feminists all over the country to denigrate the profession and its governing Council, just when they needed all possible public support for such meritorious projects as the rebuilding fund for the London Royal Veterinary College.

Professor Hobday, while unable to justify some of the admittedly ridiculous statements he himself had made, was deeply pained at McFadyean's negative attitude. However, it was only too true that the women graduates were finding it difficult to obtain employment, and McFadyean's resolution was eventually passed by thirteen votes to seven. Sir John continued to play an active part in veterinary politics to the end of his long life in 1941, but he had shot his last bolt in his opposition to women in the profession, and he did not publicly renew the subject.

The number of women in the profession grew slowly but steadily. Several obtained work by marrying male veterinary surgeons, and there were some fruitful partnerships on this basis. Most of the others set up

78

on their own and employed other women as soon as they needed assistants or *locums*. In this way employment opportunities gradually widened, although it was many years before their prospects were as good as men's. Even today a woman has to be rather better than the available men in order to obtain promotion in large organisations such as the Ministry of Agriculture or the major drug firms.

CHAPTER VII

The Old Lioness

"There is grey in your hair
Young men no longer suddenly catch their breath
When you are passing
But maybe some old gaffer mutters a blessing."

W. B. Yeats - `Broken Dreams´

By 1924 Aleen had decided to dispose finally of all her property in Ireland and sever her connections with her adopted country. She sold the house called `Fort Lyster´, from where she had practised since 1912, and also a small two-storey cottage which she had originally bought for £500. She was able to sell this for £900, which suggests there was quite a degree of post-war inflation in Ireland. The veterinary practice that she had built up with such care went eventually to a newly qualified young Irishman, Mr P. J. Healey. Soon after he took over he was presented with a batch of about a hundred colts to castrate. They had probably been accumulating for months ·during Aleen's absence. He felt quite unequal to this mammoth task, and was obliged to call in a brother practitioner to assist him.

Meanwhile Aleen had settled down in Hampshire, in the New Forest village of Plaitford, at a house called `New Lodge´. She told friends in Ireland that the New Forest was the place in England that most resembled her beloved Co. Roscommon, and that was why she had chosen it. It is ironic that now she was on the Register she made no attempt to set up in practice. At fifty-six, with a weak chest, she felt she could no longer cope with the rigours of general practice. That she had done so in her youth, and with such success, in one of the most exacting horse-breeding areas of the British Isles, was well known within the profession, and she had no need to go on proving herself. Her income was evidently sufficient for her needs, and she proceeded to enjoy herself as a country gentlewoman - but with a difference. She never forgot that she was a veterinary surgeon, and regularly attended meetings of the

National Veterinary Medical Association, being a member of both the Central Division (London) and the Southern Counties. She kept one or two horses, and she began to breed dogs - pomeranians and cocker spaniels, although she also kept odd individuals of other breeds. The cocker spaniels she developed into a breed of miniatures, which she said bred true, although the Kennel Club would not allow these as a separate breed.

She asserted that her pomeranians did not yap with the irritating shrillness characteristic of the breed, but in so far as it was true it was probably a matter of training rather than genetics. She was very strict with them, and her devotion was never without discipline. However, yapping or silent, at least one of her pomeranians reached show standard, and in September 1926 "Muffatee of Athleague" won third prize in the novice class at the Blandford and Wimborne Dog Show. It may well have been at one of these local rural occasions that Aleen was unwittingly trapped into something known as `unprofessional conduct'. She was a charismatic figure with a warm out-going personality, and it would have been all too easy for an astute young man to have got her talking. The result was half a column in *The Sunday Times* of 6th December 1925 with bold headlines:-

"The ONLY WOMAN `VET'
WORK OF SIR C. CUST'S SISTER
PROFESSION OF BIG OPPORTUNITIES"

`Our own correspondent' from Lyndhurst, gave a fairly accurate account of her career, such as could only have come from Aleen herself, who probably had no idea she was talking to a reporter. One interesting sentence read:-

"In the war she did splendid work in the chief veterinary laboratory, trying to discover the nature of the disease responsible for carrying off so many British horses."

This looks as though she really was in Captain Watson's laboratory in France during those five months in the QMAAC for which the records of the War Office are missing, believed burnt in the air raids on London in 1941. The rest of the article is taken up with Aleen's opinions of women's prospects in the profession. She thought they would do well in bacteriology and small animal practice, but while she herself had treated horses and cattle "for every possible ailment" this would be beyond the strength of most women. In conclusion the article said that she was keen on hunting and had ridden with most packs in England and Ireland, although her chief interest now lay in breeding `pocket cocker spaniels´.

At that time there were very strict rules about `advertising´, even indirectly, and Aleen was always scrupulous in observing them, but this had evidently caught her unawares. In the *Veterinary Record* of 6th February 1926 appears the following paragraph:-

> "Miss A. Cust, MRCVS, informs us that the report of an alleged interview in the *Sunday Times* of Dec. 6th last was published without her knowledge and sanction."

As well as dogs she began breeding birds, especially ornamental pheasants - golden, Amherst, and Indian. These, and some quail, she kept outside, but indoors she kept some tropical species, and eventually a whole room in her small house was given up to them.

Although not officially in practice she would always help in an emergency. Mrs Marjory Davis, who was born and brought up in the neighbourhood, vividly remembers her helping a local farmer to rescue his sow that had fallen down a disused well. Aleen got down inside with the sow, and with the farmer up above they managed to get a rope round the sow's body behind the forelegs. The farmer hauled on the rope while Aleen - up to her armpits in slurry - pushed and guided from below, and the sow was eventually heaved up and over the rim of the well to safety.

For her regular veterinary work among her own animals she usually called in Mr Facer, who practised in Southampton and was secretary to the Southern Counties Division of the NVMA. He soon became a personal friend and in her later years he was a regular visitor socially.

For a few years she lived in the village of Plaitford, but in 1927 she decided she would like somewhere more secluded, and she had a small house built to her requirements deep in the heart of the Forest, north of Bramshaw. There is a very old legend in the Forest, and I believe current in one or two other places, that if anyone can build a house at such speed that between sunset and sunrise they can get the roof on and the chimney smoking, it entitles them to various squatters' rights and privileges. I am assured by local Forestry Officers that this custom died out several centuries ago, and that it never applied to anything more than small hovels used by itinerant outlaws. However, Aleen was a born raconteuse and insisted that her new house had fulfilled these conditions, and her younger cousins listened wide-eyed and firmly believed her. While she seems to have been totally ignored by her father's family, several of her mother's relatives remained her friends, and some of the younger generation thought much of her. In contrast to her sister Ursula, who disliked children, Aleen had a warmth and friendliness that drew them to her. Her obsession with dogs and horses by no means excluded other interests, and it is said that she wrote poetry and was very artistic, as well as being an observant naturalist. Such gifts, coupled with her unusual career and the fame it had eventually brought her, must have made her a fascinating figure, especially to children brought up in more conventional circles.

Life still held some surprises for her, and soon after the new house was built a moment's negligence on her part caused a disaster. Aleen had gone out for the evening to visit friends at Plaitford. Unfortunately she had forgotten that she had left a jar of beeswax on the hob to soften. It not only softened, but melted and ran in all directions and set the little house on fire. The thatched roof was soon well alight, but fortunately neighbours saw it in time to rescue the animals, and the Fire Brigade soon arrived from Lyndhurst. But alas, there was no good water supply and they soon found themselves unable to cope with the blaze. They sent for help from Southampton, but that was nearly sixteen miles away and by the time the Southampton Brigade arrived and got the fire under control, the house was completely gutted. Fortunately the stables and outdoor kennels were separate from the house, so most of her precious animals were safe. It must have been a sad blow, but undaunted as ever, she set about having the house rebuilt as soon as possible. This time the roof was of slate and it lasted, substantially unchanged, until after Aleen's death.

Aleen's brother, Leopold, died in the spring of 1928. There is no evidence that they had had any contact since Aleen came to England and he did not mention her in his Will. Neither did Sir Charles Cust, who died in London in 1931. This is probably good evidence that her brothers and sister had completely cut her out of their lives. Sir Charles' death was noted in the *Veterinary Record*, with due condolences to Aleen, but she probably had little need of them.

She was not without local friends, however, and Mrs Darling, of Lyndhurst, remembers often driving her Aunt Annie (Miss S. A. Timson) over to Bramshaw to visit Miss Cust. Aunt Annie kept King Charles' Spaniels, and the two old ladies had much in common. Dazel Wood Corner, Miss Cust's house, was a comfortable untidy place with lots of animals flowing in and out of it. She no longer had as large a staff as when she lived in Ireland before the war, but she seems to have had a resident housekeeper companion of some sort for most of the time, while a man who lived locally did the rough work outside. She had moved with the times. She now wore breeches on horseback and rode astride, and her grey hair was cut in a `bob´, but she always changed for dinner right to the end, although this evening meal of hers was a very simple one.

Early in 1932 she spent some weeks in the West Indies, possibly on medical advice to avoid the English winter. She visited Jamaica, where she did some useful work for the Royal Society for the Prevention of Cruelty to Animals and made many friends. She came back bursting with energy, and at the June meeting of the Southern Counties Veterinary Association she described a device used in Trinidad to prevent horses slipping on the smooth asphalt roads there. This consisted of pads of rubber, cut from old motor tyres, which could be nailed on to the shoe when it was fitted, and she thought them worth a trial on British roads. Her description suggests that they may have been a more primitive version of `Gray's flexible bridge bar pad´ which was used for the same purposes in England in the thirties. At this meeting Aleen also described the use of motor exhaust gases as a painless and effective method of destroying dogs.

Later that year, in July 1932, she again went abroad, this time to France on a trip organised by the *Veterinary Journal* to visit the Alfort Veterinary School near Paris. The party numbered twenty-two, and included general practitioners, professors, and students. The leader of the party was her old friend Professor Hobday, now Principal of the Royal Veterinary College, London. By all accounts it was a crowded and memorable weekend. They spent Sunday sight-seeing, and visited Pasteur's tomb. On Monday they visited the Alfort Veterinary School - one of the oldest in Europe - and they also visited an abattoir, and had lunch at the Paris Zoological Gardens. They were particularly impressed with the museum and library at Alfort, which was much better endowed that the impoverished Royal Veterinary College, London.

It must have been just before or after this visit that Aleen called, briefly, at the London College and was introduced to the women students. There were about thirty or more of them at that time and they were very thrilled and excited to meet her. The writer was in her third year, and has a vivid memory of a handsome old lady with a beautiful voice. She was dignified, but very warm and friendly.

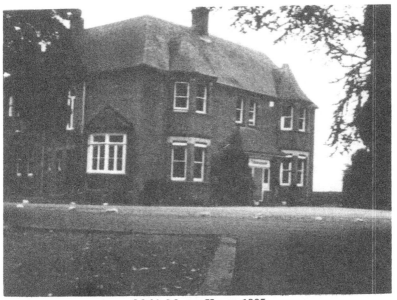

Maids Morton House, 1985

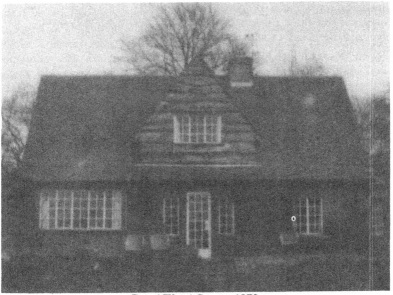

Dazel Wood Corner, 1978

By 1934 there were thirty-one women on the Veterinary Register, although not all of them had obtained gainful employment in the profession. Perhaps to boost their morale and do something to combat the prevailing prejudice against them, the Central Veterinary Society, London, decided to hold what was subsequently termed a `Ladies Night` for its meeting on 1st March 1934. Three women, Marjorie Jordan, Beatrice Lock, and Kathleen Shedlock, all of whom had been qualified for several years, were invited to read short papers. Five other women graduates were present, with several women students as visitors, and the meeting was crowded with their male colleagues, professors and other staff from the London Veterinary College. It was a most distinguished audience, but very sympathetic and friendly. The women spoke well, although none of them had enough experience to contribute much of scientific value. The issue of the *Veterinary Record* of 7th April 1934 in which this meeting was fully reported also contained a number of invited clinical articles from other women, several of whom had not been able to be present at the `Central` meeting. Among these contributions was a two-page article headed "Memories and Memos" by Aleen Cust. This was the first and last contribution of substance that Aleen made to the veterinary press after she was officially qualified. It is reproduced here in full, as being typical of her lucid, racy style, and also because it illustrates some facets of practice in the early years of the twentieth century. Her hints for emergency treatment are basically sound, and comprise the kind of useful information that is not to be found in textbooks.

"My dear Women Colleagues,

It is not my intention to write a clinical article, but rather a friendly letter in which I hope you may find a few useful tips, some learnt by bitter experience, others passed on to me by many kind men who have helped me along my stony road. I have had the *inestimable* privilege of attaining my life's ambition, I have known the world at its best in what was *then* the best country in the world (Ireland). I have also known the world at its worst, alas!

That I achieved my life's goal is due to many things - Fate, Luck, Tenacity, Heredity: the last by no means least for one of my grandmothers had the same undying passion for animals and `a way with them`. She had in her library all the known works on animal ailments suitable for the lay mind. She was the first to

86

write on the Diseases of Cats (*such* a quaint little book, long since out of print, very amateurish in its odd remedies - `Flies are very pernicious to cats. They make them thin.' is one of its sentences.) Nevertheless her favourite white Persian cat lived to be twenty-two, so her methods of cat management cannot have been so very wrong. The same cat crossed the Atlantic 18 times, as she always took it with her on her annual voyage to her villa in Madeira, and it travelled in a basket with five padlocks for great, greater, greatest security!

She was also, I believe, the first to study the breeding habits of chameleons and wrote a brochure on them. She rode after she was 80, doctored her own animals, on one occasion had six of her horses shot the same day, previous to one of her voyages, rather than run the risk of their falling into bad hands; drove with two Dalmation dogs running under her carriage and died, alas, before I knew her.

Like me, she was born many many years too soon. Had she lived later she might have been the first woman veterinary surgeon and I would have been her humble follower. I treasure now some of her beautiful shagreen cases of instruments, many of them ivory handled and more suited to human surgery as it was then practised.

She at least would have understood the urge that was in me from earliest childhood. When asked what I wanted: `To be a whipper-in to hounds, an M.F.H., a rough rider', a *vet* was my reply ever and always.

I remember, when a child, collecting sea-bleached bones washed up by the tide, hiding a boxful of them under my bed, sitting up in my nighty when supposed to be asleep, wondering if I would ever be able (like the great Professor Owen) to piece them together and to know what animal they came from. But one bad day my treasures were discovered and thrown away and again I was in disgrace.

Instead of locks of human hair I kept locks of horses' and dogs' hair in the little lockets then fashionable which aunts, etc., had given me to keep their own locks in. I don't remember not owning pets of some sort - before I could walk I insisted on riding our big Newfoundland dog rather than go in my pram and I can still remember the feel of his shaggy neck as I clutched it, pillowing my face therein; my first very own pony "Taffy", a Welsh strawberry roan newly clipped, bolting, to my great

87

delight; the proud moment of my first side saddle and, Oh, the first riding habit with its little trousers! (no jodhpurs in those days.) I was then about six; driving our donkey "Robin" in a new three-wheeled wicker chair bought for my mother, Robin bolting as he was traced too short and the front wheel touched his heels, I was thrown out on the gravel drive when the whole thing upset, knocking out some of my teeth (luckily the baby ones) my old Irish nanny spending the afternoon hunting for them, with I suppose, a view to sticking them in again!

But to later days.

In a rough country practice in Ireland, such as mine was, one had to rely on one's own resourcefulness to an extent undreamed of by the town practitioner of these days in his perfectly equipped premises with everything at hand. My work was chiefly with horses and cattle owned by the most horse-loving, horse-knowing, keenly critical people in the world - people intolerant of bluff or eyewash, helpful, plucky, keen on their animals, ready to carry out one's instructions regardless of time or trouble if only "the baste can be saved, your honour". But alas! too often they had exhausted their own charms and philtres before giving up hope and sending for me. "How long is she bad Pat?" "Well now I won't be telling your honour a lie but she's bad this week and more" (the little more and how much it was!).

But I'd never stop telling all the tales and wondrous remedies they used.

Probably most of you will specialise in small animals, but those who are going to rough it may find some useful suggestions in this bran-pie of mine.

A pair of pillowcases filled with hot dry bran heated in a bucket till it just doesn't burn is very useful in pneumonia of the horse. Keep two sets going and change hourly.

If a horse will not swallow a drench pour a little down one nostril - but this is dangerous, mind.

Don't stand in front of a horse with tetanus when you are going to shoot him, as he will fall right forward.

A large funnel and a bit of tubing (even bicycle tubing if you can find a stiff piece) makes a very efficient enema apparatus in an emergency.

A pair of fire tongs with a block of wood between is far better than *no* gag with the kind of horse who likes chewing on his own doubled-up tongue and your hand.

A wisp of hay or even grass tied into a knot of your castrating rope prevents the knot from jamming.

A firing iron softens the hoof if you have a Smith's operation to do on a very hard and thick wall. But be quick to follow the hot iron with your knife.

If anyone has seen a horse with `head staggers' wearing an open bridle I would be very interested to hear it, as I believe the discarding of blinkers in such cases acts as a specific preventive.

If a horse will not lead into a stable, try a longer rope and march ahead *without looking back at him*. This often works better than trying to back him in.

If out hunting a horse gets cast in a narrow ditch, get hold of a stirrup leather, iron and all (two if needs be) and loop them over the far fetlocks, pulling him over till he can grip the lowest side of the ditch.

If no funnel is available and you want to pour from a large bucket into a small bottle, grip the bucket with your knees, lay the flat of your thumbs along the rim and let your thumbs form a channel for the water.

A hypodermic injection of strychnine plus, of course, demulcents is worth trying in impaction of the oesophagus of the horse before resorting to more heroic measures, but be careful if the animal is a cow. I killed one once with half a grain, but she'd have died anyway.

Nux vomica in large doses orally combined with other stimulants will often bring away a putrid placenta from a cow, and it's a much less unpleasant way than by manual manipulation, I assure you! But if you *must* remove it by hand, waterproof your arm with, say, vaseline impregnated with ol. eucalyptus one in eight. Otherwise they will be able to run a drag with you for days after!

And now we are on cows and you've forgotten your milk fever outfit, and, of course, have no calcium sandoz, etc.: borrow a bicycle pump, take out the valve, boil it, use it as a teat syphon, and pump away.

A prolapsed uterus or vagina can be retained by ordinary butcher skewers with tape or string zig-zagged if all your West's clamps are in use or left at home. Every house has these. Talking of this, if you have to perform tracheotomy to prevent straining afterwards, don't tie her by the neck chain but by a rope round her

89

horns or with a halter if she is a Polled breed. Otherwise she will tear out the tube.

Few cows will kick if the tail is held on a level with or rather above the back. Twisting the tail round the hock is also a useful dodge, but do not let the holder of it be too zealous or he may pull the skin off the tail as you do to a fox's brush. This happened to me once, but mercifully it was the cow's owner who had the tail.

The screwdriver of your car outfit is quite useful to puncture post-pharangeal abscesses or in white heifer disease if your finger nail is not a very hard one, and it is not so apt to retire inside a restless patient as is a Syme's knife.

I take a great interest in all of you and in your careers and your successes, and my wish for you is that you, my Women Colleagues, may all feel as I do after a lifetime - that the profession you have chosen is *the* Best Profession in the World.

Goodbye now; success and happiness to you all and may you have `the lucky hand´.

Yours sincerely,

Aleen Cust, MRCVS

Dazel Wood Corner, Bramshaw, Lyndhurst.
March 25th 1934"

In place of the usual brief editorial this issue of the *Veterinary Record* contains a rather long `contributed´ but unsigned article on women in the profession - past, present and future. It is unctuously complimentary about Miss Cust, gives a benevolent pat on the head for all the rest, especially Madeline Oyler, who had a particularly brilliant academic career, and suggests that women are admirably suited to tedious routine work, which a woman will perform more conscientiously than a man might. To a modern graduate this might seem comically patronising, but it was a healthy advance from the position of the ferocious McFadyean.

Of more interest to modern readers is the full-page photograph in the same issue of Aleen Cust in academic dress. It became her admirably, the watered silk facings gleaming against her plain tailor-made costume beneath the gown. The velvet doctor's cap - more elaborate than anything she normally wore on her head - gave her added dignity. The strong features and faraway gaze have a touch of sadness in them, and the hands are unusually large and powerful. She stands very upright, but curiously alert, as if she might move off out of the picture at any moment. This studio portrait is almost certainly the source of an enlarged charcoal drawing, made at the behest of the Society of Women Veterinary Surgeons in 1965, and now hanging in the RCVS Library at Belgrave Square. This is quite a good likeness, but the artist has been unable to resist the temptation to pretty it up and tone it down. The hands are smaller, and the strength of the face is diminished to petulance, but for those who would seek the true spirit of this woman the photograph is there, in the *Veterinary Record* of 1934.

As the years passed Aleen gradually became more frail and did not venture out so often, although she still drove her own car, a very old and noisy Trojan, probably of about 1930 vintage. Her mind dwelling on the past she began thinking of Bertram Widdrington, to whom she had been briefly engaged in 1904. He had risen to the rank of Brigadier General, and on retirement from the army he settled in Buckinghamshire in the village of Maids Moreton, with his wife and two sons. His wife's mother also lived with them. He still owned Newton Hall in Northumberland, and visited it regularly for the shooting. His mother, Cecilia Widdrington, was still alive, and it was possibly from Cecilia that Aleen learned of his whereabouts. She determined to look him up, and in 1935 she arrived, unheralded, on his doorstep one summer afternoon. Bertram and his wife received her very kindly, and the two boys were much intrigued to learn of the connection. Francis, the young son, was a lad of fifteen and very like his father. Aleen would have known Bertram very well when he was that age, and the resemblance must have been quite startling for her. She took an immediate fancy to Francis, and told Bertram that as she had no children of her own she thought of making Francis her heir. She seems to have given them the impression that she was a woman of considerable wealth and property, and young Francis was suitably impressed at the prospect of this inheritance.

However, back in her home she seems to have thought better of it, and the Will she drew up in the course of the next year does not mention him. Perhaps the sight of Bertram, elderly and balding although very well preserved, was something of a disillusionment, and his comfortable circumstances in the midst of a loving family made any bequest she might make somewhat superfluous. It would have been a romantic gesture from someone who, from a conventional point of view, was an also-ran in the all-important marriage stakes.

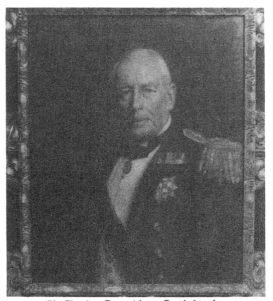

Sir Charles Cust, Aleen Cust's brother

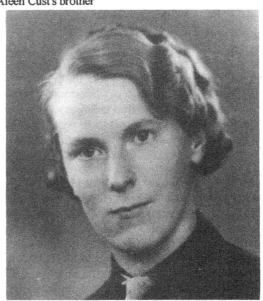

Pat Williams, MRCVS, circa 1935

In the summer of 1935 a quiet girl, who loved horses and dogs, qualified as a veterinary surgeon from the London Veterinary College. Petronel Louisa Williams - Pat to her friends - had slogged her way through the four year course, beginning in Liverpool but spending the last two years in London. She loved the work, and was eminently suited to it, but there seemed to be no hope of her getting a job. For months she kept applying for all the jobs advertised, but many of the advertisers did not even bother to reply to her application. Principal Hobday, now Sir Frederick Hobday, had lost the illusions of his early euphoria and was dismayed and irritated at the procession of forlorn women graduates who remained unemployed and whom he was unable to help find work. Pat felt her hard-won skills slipping from her through disuse, and decided on bold action. She wrote to Miss Cust asking for advice.

Something in this letter must have stirred Aleen's memories of her own early struggles and the desperate determination with which she tackled them. She invited Pat to Dazel Wood Corner and offered her a job. She made it clear that this was not professional work, being merely to help look after all her birds and animals, but she hinted that it might lead to something more.

So for six months Pat lived in the shadow of greatness in Miss Cust's household. She mucked out kennels, groomed the dogs and horses, chopped up meal worms for the small tropical birds, and acted as general dog's body. The old lady was kind, but very exacting and autocratic. Pat's adored old poodle - from whom she was never normally separated - was banished to an outside kennel. There were compensations, however, permission to exercise the horses ranking high among them. There was an old favourite cob that Miss Cust had ridden until recently. Now they were both of them somewhat infirm, and it was while Pat was with her that this old horse eventually had to be destroyed, which must have been a very sad occasion. But Aleen still had a Welsh pony stallion, and Pat was delighted to be allowed to ride him. Aleen warned her that he had mares in the Forest whom he regarded as his own, and he was apt to try to rejoin them, but Pat evidently managed him to Miss Cust's satisfaction.

In March 1936 Aleen took Pat to a meeting of the Southern Counties Veterinary Association at Winchester, and introduced her to other members. Perhaps Aleen remembered how helpful it was to her when Willie Byrne had used his famous charm to introduce his young protegee at the Irish veterinary meetings. The piquant difference was that whereas Aleen had been doing veterinary work although not legally qualified, here was Pat, impeccably on the Register, but working as a kennelmaid.

But Pat's hard work and Miss Cust's scheming on her behalf eventually bore fruit and later in the year Mr Facer of Southampton took her on as *locum tenens* when he was on holiday. This was her first real chance, and Pat evidently came through with flying colours. The ice had been broken and other temporary jobs followed, including one with Frank Chambers, a practitioner of considerable prestige in Wolverhampton, who recognised her ability and befriended her thereafter. Within a year Pat had purchased the nucleus of a small practice in Stafford, which she ran successfuly for some years until the second World War disrupted it.

Before Pat left Dazel Wood Corner Miss Cust gave her four veterinary textbooks. One on `Castration´ was written by Hobday and inscribed "with the author's compliments, Sept. 1914". The other bears Aleen's signature and the dates 1900 for `Muller's Diseases of the Dog´, 1903 for Dollar's `Operative Technique´ and 1904 for Captain Hayes' `Veterinary Notes for Horse Owners´. These are still among Pat's most treasured possessions, and Aleen's signatures on them are almost the only specimens of her hand-writing that survive. Miss Cust also gave Pat some veterinary instruments which she used later on in her own practice.

After Pat's departure Aleen seems to have drooped a little. She did not attend the September meeting of the Southern Counties Veterinary Association, but sent her apologies. The onset of winter depressed her, and her doctor thought she would do better in a warmer climate, so she planned to spend three months with friends in Jamaica. True to form she had no intention of relaxing on a chaise longue, but, assuming that the sun would give her back her energy, she planned a tour of the island on horseback. Captain G. O. Rushie Grey, a veterinary surgeon in Jamaica, promised to arrange this for her.

Before sailing she prudently tidied up her affairs and made a final codicil to her Will on the 2nd December 1936. This Will was most complicated and detailed. She wished to be buried in Bramshaw churchyard, near her home, the funeral to be as inexpensive as possible and only horse-drawn vehicles to be used for it. She left all her dogs and other livestock, kennels and kennel appliances, to Miss Mary Elisabeth Simms, then living in Ireland, who had lived with Miss Cust in Hampshire from 1930 to 1933. Bequests of money - from one hundred to several hundred pounds - were left to a number of other people, some local but mostly in Ireland. She left all her silver "which formerly belonged to the late Major Augustus Blair Mayne" to Phyllis Lady Moore, wife of Sir Frederick Moore of Dublin. Sir Frederick was famous as a veterinary historian of military matters.

94

A more substantial sum of £3,000 was to be invested in trust to provide an income for Mrs Georgina Bagot, of Athleague, Roscommon, and her son Captain Ted Bagot. The Bagots had been her nearest neighbours in Athleague. Next came the legacy by which her name is most often remembered within the profession. She left the RCVS £5,000 to be invested, and the income used for a scholarship in veterinary research. It was to be awarded from time to time as the Council of the RCVS thought fit, and to be called the Aleen Cust Research Scholarship. The scholars could be of any age, but must be "natural born English, Scottish, Welsh or Irish men or women". She expressed a wish that "in deciding between candidates for the scholarship who are otherwise in their opinion of equal merit the Council shall as between men and women give preference to women". For one who had seen such bigotted prejudice and discrimination against women all her life this showed an admirable magnanimity and common sense. Today, owing to recent inflation, the legacy is much diminished in value, and it is usually merged with others, but the details of it were still printed in one of the appendices to the RCVS register of 1985.

She also left £100 to endow a dog kennel at the Royal Veterinary College, London, in memory of her miniature cocker spaniels. It was to be suitably inscribed with a favourite quotation:- "I freely admit that the best of my fun I owe it to horse and hound". Unfortunately the exigencies of rebuilding, provision for disinfection, and other factors of modern design made this bequest too complicated to fulfil in modern times, but it was a pleasant thought.

Her house, and the residue of her estate was left in trust for Mary Elisabeth Simms, and after her death to the British Trust for Ornithology. In the original Will the residue of her estate went eventually to Captain Ted Bagot, but the codicil of December 1936 changed this and gave it to her cousin's son, Commander Arthur Grey Skipwith. This codicil gave £100 to the British Trust for Ornithology (which was a memorial to Lord Grey of Falloden) and Aleen's gift was in memory of Lord Grey's wife, Dorothy, who was the elder daughter of the Widdringtons, and Bertram's sister. In this clause of the Will she described Dorothy, who had died in 1906, as "the greatest friend of my life".

Commander Skipwith confessed with some amusement that the residue of her estate, by the time it reached him, was practically non-existent, which was hardly surprising in view of all these thoughtful bequests, but he realised how much the old lady must have enjoyed planning it all, and her last minute thought for one of her own family is rather touching.

So she set sail for Jamaica with her mind at ease, and it so happened that she was never to return.

CHAPTER VIII

Death in Jamaica

"Sleep; and if life was bitter to thee, pardon,
if sweet, give thanks; thou hast no more to live."

Algernon Charles Swinburne - `Ave atque Vale`

Aleen arrived in Jamaica on the morning of the 5th January 1937, intending to return to England on the 7th April. She stayed at the house of Mr Frank Cundall, another veterinary surgeon with whom she was friendly, and she intended to set off next morning on her riding tour. Instead she suffered a severe heart attack that very night. She recovered remarkably well, but was confined to her room for about ten days. After that she was able to go for drives but unfit for anything more strenuous. However, on the evening of Thursday, the 28th January, she felt much better and arranged to leave the Cundall's house to go and stay with some other friends for a few more days recuperation.

Next morning, Friday the 29th, while she was packing up her belongings, the Cundall's maid came and told her that the family dog had scratched at a wart and it was bleeding, and please could she look at it. The old war-horse in her leapt into battle. She found the offending blood vessel and ligated it, thus stopping the bleeding. She then improvised a cardboard collar to prevent the dog interfering with the wound, after which she collapsed. A doctor arrived within twenty minutes, but he said she must have died immediately. Despite the shock to her hosts all realised that it was as she would have wished to go - working in her chosen profession and completing a satisfactory case. She was just eight days short of her sixty-ninth birthday.

Bibliography

Chapter I

p.1.   *The Cat. Its history diseases and management.* The Hon.
        Lady Mary Anne Cust. Published by Dranes, London.
        1880.
p.5.   Interview with Messrs J. and W. Connery, Cordangan
        Manor estate, June 7th 1981.
        The *Tipperary Free Press & Clonmel General Advertiser.*
        Tuesday 5/3/1878. `Death of Sir Leopold Cust´.

Chapter II

p.11.   *Who's Who* 1929-1944, p. 322.
        Shrewsbury Chronicle 4/8/1893, p. 5. `Death of Mr
        Brownlow Orlando Cust´.
p.12.   *Veterinary Journal* 1897, vol. 45, p. 354.
p.13.   *Veterinary Record* 14/4/1934, vol. 14, p. 416.
p.15.   Ibid. 10/8/1935, vol. 15, p. 932.
        Ibid. 15/5/1937, vol. 49, p. 630.
p.16.   Ibid. 24/4/1897, vol. 9, p. 609.
p.19.   Ibid. 15/5/1897, vol. 9, p. 649.
        Ibid. 22/5/1897, vol. 9, p. 667.
p.20.   Ibid. 5/6/1897, vol. 9, p. 692.
        Ibid. 12/6/1897, vol. 9, p. 693.
p.21.   Ibid. 1/5/1897, vol. 9, p. 627.
p.22.   Ibid. 30/10/1897, vol. 9, p. 245.
        Ibid. 22/1/1898, vol. 10, pp. 409, 411.
p.23.   Ibid. 14/4/1934, vol. 14, p. 416.

Chapter III

p.25.   *Veterinary Record* 25/5/1889, vol. 1, p. 582.
p.27.   Ibid. 30/10/1897, vol. 10, pp. 242-244.
p.28.   Ibid. 27/1/1900, vol. 12, p. 423.
p.29.   Correspondence with the Revd. Father Gerard Dolan, Diocesan
        Secretary, St. Mary's, Sligo.

	Interview with Mr Frank White of Castlestrange, 10/6/1981.
p.30.	Cecilia Widdrington's diary, courtesy of Captain A. J. Baker-Cresswell.
	Veterinary News 24/9/1910, vol. 7, p. 542.
p.33.	*Veterinary Record* 23/6/1900, vol. 12, p. 742.
p.34.	Ibid. 10/10/1903, vol. 16, p. 220.
	Ibid. 16/4/1904, vol. 16, pp. 656, 797.
p.35.	Ibid. 27/8/1904, vol. 17, p. 125.
	Ibid. 11/3/1905, vol. 17, p. 577.
p.37.	Ibid. 2/9/1905, vol. 18, p. 159.
	Ibid. 30/9/1905, vol. 18, pp. 105, 159, 229, 241.
	Ibid. 14/10/1905, vol. 18, p. 254.
p.38.	*Irish Times* 12/2/1906.
	Veterinary News 24/2/1906, vol. 3, p. 129.

Chapter IV

p.39.	*Connaught Champion* 4/11/1905. Report of Galway County Council meeting.
	Veterinary Record 11/11/1905, vol. 18, pp. 327, 342, 343.
	Ibid. 18/11/1905, vol. 18, p. 356.
p.41.	Ibid. 31/8/1907, vol. 20, p. 155.
p.43.	Ibid. 11/11/1905, vol. 18, p. 346. Quoted from *Ballinasloe Western News*.
	Veterinary News 4/11/1905, vol. 12, p. 549.
	Ibid. 11/11/1905, vol. 12, p. 564.
	Veterinary Journal, November 1905, vol. 12, p. 267 Editorial; p. 325 Personal; p. 384 Correspondence.
	Connaught Champion 23/6/1906, Council Proceedings.
	Veterinary Record 19/5/1906, vol. 18, p. 826. Quoted from *Irish Independent* 16/5/1906.
	Veterinary Record 6/10/1906, vol. 19, p. 199.
	Connaught Champion 3/2/1906, Council Proceedings.
	Veterinary Record 14/9/1907, vol. 20, p. 176.
p.45.	Ibid. 12/10/1906, vol. 20, p. 263.
	Ibid. 9/11/1907, vol. 20, p. 335. Quoted from *The Leader*.
	Ibid. 17/4/1909, vol. 21, p. 723.
	Ibid. 4/11/1909, vol. 22, p. 311.
p.46.	Ibid. 4/11/1909, vol. 22, p. 314.

	Ibid. 23/4/1910, vol. 22, p. 706.
	Roscommon Messenger, 23/4/1910.
	Veterinary Record 30/4/1910, vol. 22, p. 708.
	Veterinary Journal, May 1910, vol. 17, p. 245.
p.47.	Interview with Mr James Cox of Athleague, 12/6/1981.
	Interview with Mr James Waldron of Athleague, 12/6/1981.
p.48.	Correspondence with Mr John Evans, MRCVS, 1985.
p.49.	*Veterinary Record* 29/10/1910, vol. 23, p. 275.
	Ibid. 9/9/1911, vol. 24, p. 171.
	Ibid. 1/11/1913, vol. 26, p. 288.
p.50.	Ibid. 18/10/1913, vol. 26, p. 247.
	Ibid. 13/12/1913, vol. 26, pp. 369, 381.
p.51.	*Daily Mail*, 24/12/1912. Girton's Girl's appeal to High Court.
p.52.	*Veterinary Record* 28/2/1914, vol. 26, p. 568.
	Ibid. 8/8/1914, vol. 27, p. 97.

Chapter V

p.53.	*Veterinary Record* 29/5/1897, vol. 9, p. 674.
	The Horse and the War by Captain Sidney Galtrey. Published by *Country Life* 1918.
p.54.	*Journal of the Royal Artillery* 1950, vol. 77, pp. 213-222. Lt. Gen. Sir George McMunn, KCB, KCSI, DSO.
	The Army Veterinary Service in War by Major Gen. Sir John Moore, KCMG, CB, FRCS. Published by H. W. Brown, London 1921.
p.57.	*Our Servant the Horse* by Major Gen. Sir J. Moore, KCMG, CB, FRCS. Published by H. W. Brown, London 1931.
	Veterinary Record 21/12/1918, vol. 31, p. 205.
p.59.	Tuam Quarter Sessions 13/1/1915. Cust v. Fallon.
p.60.	Public Records Office, Kew. W.O. 95-69 Diary of the Director of Remount Services (Brig. Gen. Sir Francis Sudlow Garratt), 16/11/1916.
p.61.	Public Records Office, Kew. W.O. 95-69 War Diary of the Director of Veterinary Services (Brig. Gen. Sir J. Moore), 1/1/1917, 8/1/1917, 19/9/1917, 16/11/1917.
p.62.	Ministry of Defence, Hayes, Middlesex. Correspondence, 1981.

Public Records Office, Kew. W.O. 95-85. War Diary of
Controller, Rouen QMAAC (Name unknown, initials
unidentified), 13/2/1918.
Service with the Army by Dame Helen Gwynne-Vaughan,
Chief Controller WAAC. Published by Hutchinson 1917.
Interview with Mrs Madeline Curtis (née Coppin) of Romford,
13/8/1984.
p.63.   Public Records Office, Kew. W.O. 95-85. War Diary of Area
Controller Rouen QMAAC, 7/7/1918.
p.64.   Interviews and correspondence with Commander Arthur Grey
Skipwith, R.N. of Twyford, Winchester, 1982-86.

Chapter VI

p.65.   *Veterinary Record* 10/7/1915, vol. 28, pp. 11, 18.
p.66.   Ibid. 31/7/1915, vol. 28, p. 54. Quoted from *The Animals'
Guardian.*
         The Times 22/4/1915.
p.67.   *Veterinary Record* 1/2/1918, vol. 30, p. 268.
         Ibid. 19/4/1919, vol. 31, pp. 369, 373.
         Ibid. 19/4/1919, vol. 31, pp. 373, 375.
p.69.   Ibid. 18/10/1919, vol. 32, p. 174.
         Ibid. 25/10/1919, vol. 32, p. 184.
p.70.   The Sex Disqualification (Removal) Act 1919, 9 & 10 Geo. 5
c. 71.
p.71.   *Veterinary Record* 24/1/1920, vol. 32, pp. 347, 352.
         Ibid. 14/2/1920, vol. 32, p. 392.
         Ibid. 20/8/1921, vol. 33, p. 652.
p.71.   Interviews and correspondence with Mrs E. G. Taylor (née
Knight), MRCVS, BSc. 28/7/1981 et seq.
p.74.   *Veterinary Record* 21/10/1922, vol. 34, p. 789.
         Ibid. 28/10/1922, vol. 34, p. 807.
         Ibid. 23/12/1922, vol. 34, pp. 952-4.
         Ibid. 6/1/1923, vol. 35, pp. 6, 8.
         Ibid. 13/1/1923, vol. 35, p. 21. Quoted from *The Field.*
         The Field 30/12/1922.
p.75.   *The Daily Chronicle* 21/12/1922.
         The Daily News 21/12/1922.
         The Daily Telegraph 21/12/1922.
         The Irish Times 21/12/1922.

The Times 21/12/1922, pp. 3, 14.
Veterinary Journal, January 1923, vol. 79, p. 7.
Veterinary Record 3/3/1923, vol. 35, p. 153.
Ibid. 10/3/1923, vol. 35, p. 177.
Ibid. 31/3/1923, vol. 35, p. 229.
Ibid. 7/4/1923, vol. 35, p. 244.
Ibid. 2/6/1923, vol. 35, p. 399.
p.76.   Ibid. 27/10/1923, vol. 35, p. 783.
Ibid. 10/11/1923, vol. 35, p. 827.
Ibid. 5/1/1924, vol. 36, p. 15.
p.77.   Ibid. 4/5/1929, vol. 41, p. 383.

Chapter VII

p.81.   Lymington and South Hants Chronicle 2/6/1927, p. 6.
           Ibid 9/6/1927, p. 3 (picture)
           Sunday Times 6/12/1925.
p.82.   Veterinary Record 6/2/1926, vol. 38, p. 138.
p.83.   Interview with Mrs Marjory Davis of Bramshaw, 14/6/1985.
           Interview with Mr F. G. Sturney of Lyndhurst, retired member
               of the local Fire Brigade, 9/10/1985.
           Veterinary Record 24/1/1931, vol. 43, p. 104
           Correspondence with Mrs C. Darling of Lyndhurst, 9/10/1985.
p.84.   Veterinary Record 17/9/1932, vol. 44, p. 1135.
           Veterinary Journal Sept. 1932, vol. 88, p. 395.
p.86.   Veterinary Record 7/4/1934, vol. 46, p. 361 et seq.
pp. 90,91. Interviews with Captain Francis Widdrington of Newton Hall,
               Northumberland, 1982 & 1986.
           Interview with Mr W. Franklin of Maids Moreton, 27/9/1985.
               (Chauffeur to the late Brig. Gen. Bertram Widdrington).
p.93.   Extensive correspondence and discussions with Mrs P. L.
               Hewlett, MRCVS (née Williams), 1980 et seq.
           Veterinary Record 21/3/1936, vol. 48, p. 367.
p.95.   Correspondence with Mr Albert Siggins of Castlestrange,
               Roscommon.
p.97.   Veterinary Record 6/2/1937, vol. 49, p. 167.
           Ibid. 27/2/1937, vol. 49, p. 274.

Index

Abbeville, 60, 62
Aleen Cust Research Scholarship, 95
Alfort Veterinary School, 84
Anderson, Elizabeth Garrett, 12, 66
Anglo-Irish War, 72
Animals' Guardian, 66
Army Veterinary Corps, 57, 61
Arnold & Sons, 45
Athleague, 46, 47, 72
Aveston, J. J., 75
Bagot, Mrs Georgina, 95
Bagot, Ted, 95
Ballinasloe, 49
Ballinasloe Western News, 42
Ballygar, 29
Barker, Captain J. R., 77
Barrymore, Lord, 1
Beale, Miss, 12
Bebb, Gwyneth Marjorie, 51, 52, 65
Belgian Jockey Club, 13
Bell, E. A., 51
Birkbeck, Major General Sir William, 53
Blandford & Wimborne Dog Show, 81
Boer War, 54
Bowes, Colonel H. G., 75
Bradford, Earl of, 1, 12
Bradley, Professor O. Charnock, 15
Bramshaw, 82, 83, 94
`Brickbat´, 53, 54
Bridgeman, Charles Orlando, 3
British Jockey Club, 13
British Trust for Ornithology, 95
British Veterinary Association, 28, 71
Broad, W. T. D., 71
Brownlow, Lord, 1
Buss, Miss, 12
Byrne, William Augustine, 12, 24, 25, 28, 29, 32-35, 37, 43, 45, 46, 49, 72, 93

Cambridge University, 20
Cameron, Mr, 45
Cameron, Sir Charles, 46
Canadian Army Veterinary Corps, 61
Canadian Veterinary profession, 63
Castlestrange, 25, 47
Castration operation, 27, 41, 48, 94
Central Veterinary Association of Ireland, 27, 28, 32, 49, 50
Central Veterinary Society (London) - (Division of the B.V.A.), 37, 75,
    81, 86
Chambers, Frank, 94
Chameleons, 87
Chylous Ascites, 46
Cocker Spaniels, 47, 81, 82, 95
Congress, Annual, of B.V.A. & predecessors:- Dublin 1900, 28, 32;
    Windermere 1903, 34; Dublin 1904, 35; Buxton 1905, 37
Congresses, International Veterinary:- 8th, Budapest 1905, 37; 10th,
    London 1914, 52
Corbet, Lady, 59
Cordangan Manor, 1
Cottesmore, 15
Cox, James, 47
Cundall, Frank, 97
Curtis, Mrs Madeline (nee Coppin), 63
Cust - other members of the family:-
    Brownlow Orlando (brother), 11, 12
    Sir Charles Leopold (brother), 6, 8, 23, 75, 81, 83
    Lady Charlotte Sobieske Isabel (née Bridgeman) (mother), 1, 3, 6, 11,
        13, 22, 59
    Sir Edward (grandfather), 3
    Sir Leopold (father), 1, 3-8, 75
    Leopold Peregrine Edward (brother), 1, 59, 83
    Lady Mary Anne (née Boode) (grandmother), 1, 86, 87
    Percy Edmund Leopold (brother), 11
    Miss Ursula (sister), 3, 59, 75, 83
Cust Rope Release Hobbles, 45
Custance, Henry, 13
Dalling, Major, 57
Darling, Mrs, 83
Davis, Mrs Marjory, 82
Dawes, H. J., 34

Dazel Wood Corner, 82, 83, 93
De Valera, 72
Dollar, J. A. W., 19, 42, 94
Dublin Children's Hospital, 47
Dublin Horse Show, 32
Dublin Veterinary College, 28, 35, 71
Easter Rising, 72
Edinburgh Court of Sessions, 22
Edinburgh (Dick) Veterinary College, 13, 15
Edinburgh University, 13
English, Miss, 49
Euthanasia, Canine, 84
Facer, John, 82
Farriers' strike 1897, 55
`Fellow from the Country`, 20
Felton, 8
Field, The, 74
Fort Lyster, 47, 80
Galway County Council, 29, 39-41, 43
Garnett, F. W., 66, 69, 70
Garratt, Brigadier General F. S., 54, 60
Garrett-Anderson, Dr Elizabeth, 12, 66
George V, King, 1, 23, 57
Glanders, 55
Glasgow Veterinary College, 16, 78
Gooch, F. L., 35
Gray's flexible bridge bar pad, 84
Greig, Thomas H., 50
Grey, G. O. Rushie, 94
Grey, Viscount, later Lord Grey of Falloden, 8, 95
Gwynne-Vaughan, Dame Helen, 62
Hayes, Captain, *Veterinary Notes for Horse Owners*, 94
`Head staggers`, 89
Healey, P. J., 80
Henry IV, King, 51
Herriot, James, 30
Highland and Agricultural Society of Scotland, 66
Hoare, Wallis, 44
Hobday, Professor Sir Frederick, 37, 48, 49, 57, 77, 78, 84, 93, 94
Howard, P. J., 49
Irish Central Veterinary Society, 27, 28, 37, 49

Moore, Lady Phyllis, 94
`Muffattee of Athleague´, 81
Muller's *Diseases of the Dog*, 94
Mulvey, W. J., 16, 17, 69-71
Murray, Dr Flora, 66
National Veterinary Medical Association (see British Veterinary Association)
New Forest, 80, 82, 83
New Lodge, Plaitford, 80
Newton Hall, 8, 23, 30, 91
Newton, Sir Isaac, 1
New Veterinary College, Edinburgh, 10, 28, 33, 75
Nightingale, Florence, 12
North British Agriculturalist, 33
North Salop Yeomanry, 11
Oyler, Madeline, 90
Plaitford, Hants., 82, 83
Pomeranian dogs, 81
Pritchard, Professor, 17, 19
Queen Mary's Army Auxillary Corps, 62, 63
Quorn, 15
Reading Agricultural College, 67, 71
Remount Service, 60, 61
`Roaring´ in horses, 48, 49
Roman Catholic Church and clergy, 5, 29, 46, 48
Roscommon, 25, 27, 59, 80
Roscommon Messenger, 46
Rouen QMAAC, 79, 80
Royal Army Veterinary Corps, 57
Royal College of Veterinary Surgeons, 16, 21, 39-42, 49-53, 65-69, 74, 77, 78, 95
Royal Counties Veterinary Association (later a Division of the NVMA and BVA), 19, 71
Royal Society for the Prevention of Cruelty to Animals, 54, 61, 84
Royal Veterinary College, London, 25, 75, 77, 78, 84, 86
Sansaw Hall, Shrewsbury, 6
Sex Disqualification (Removal) Act 1919, 70, 71, 75
Share-Jones, Professor J., 66, 67
Shedlock, Kathleen, 86
Shrewsbury Chronicle, 11
Simms, Mary Elisabeth, 94, 95

For Product Safety Concerns and Information please contact our EU
representative GPSR@taylorandfrancis.com Taylor & Francis Verlag GmbH,
Kaufingerstraße 24, 80331 München, Germany

Printed and bound by CPI Group (UK) Ltd, Croydon, CR0 4YY
01/05/2025
01858541-0001